My Crazy Mind
My Life With Bipolar Disorder

Based on Actual Events

Dominick Delarosso

Dominick Delarosso

DEDICATION

I dedicate this book to all the wonderful Doctors and Psychiatrists and the medical community who help so many people who suffer from bipolar and other mental illnesses. They are wonderful. Also I dedicate this book to all who suffer from bipolar disorder. My hope is that this book will bring many people in for help dealing with this mental illness. I dedicate this book to the many people who seek and find Jesus and except Him as their savior. This book would have never been written if it weren't for my belief in Jesus.

Dominick Delarosso

ACKNOWLEDGEMENTS:

First and foremost I thank Renee Klatt for all her love, caring and understanding. Without her this project would have never come to fruition. I also thank Kay Gonzalez a wonderful woman and the best editor anyone could ask for. I thank Paula for all her love and caring and giving me the benefit of doubt even when I did not deserve it. I thank Pat for her love, caring and understanding even when I put her through hell.

Table of Contents

September, 2010

Well, here I am in a mission in Portland, Oregon. It is cold and raining outside, but I guess I should be grateful; it could be worse. I could be under a bridge, in a doorway, or perhaps in jail or prison. I feel so depressed at times that I want to end my life, but for some reason I cannot bring myself to do it. Maybe God has other plans for me. How often I have hated myself for not having the courage to end the pain and loneliness that I feel; and at times, I feel completely hopeless.

I have thought about jumping from one of the many tall buildings in Portland, or throwing myself in front of the Max light rail or a big rig. Several times, I have come within seconds of actually doing it. On top of that, the unimaginable came true. I have to leave the mission because I have exceeded my allotted time there, which is thirty days. My shoes have holes in them, and my feet are wet. Where will I go? What will I do now?

What bothers me most is I see all these other people who seem to have a normal life, and I do not. I see them going out go to lunch and dinner or movie, or I see them enjoying happy hour, and I cannot. I watch them buy nice things, and I remember how I used to do that. I had a nice car and a motorcycle. I lived in a beautiful home with a wonderful woman.

We had a great life together, aside from my bipolar condition and the crazy decisions that I made, which caused me to lose everything in my life. When I explain to people about my life, I usually will tell them it is as if a nuclear bomb went off in the middle of my life and destroyed everything. To this, add loneliness, because being homeless is very lonely. The only people am around are other homeless persons in the missions and in the food lines. The food lines are long and the food will keep a person alive, but that is about all. I could have spent all day just getting something to eat; but I could not do that as I had to find a job; therefore, I only ate only once a day.

There is a restaurant here called Sisters of the Road Café for the homeless. If you have money, they will sell you a meal for a dollar and a half. If you do not, then you can work it off. They always have rice and beans with gravy and cornbread. They also have a different meal to choose from, usually soup and cornbread, for the same price. The nice thing about it is that one is treated like a person, not like a homeless bum. We have to wait in long lines to get in inside. Once inside, we sit at a table and one of the workers, another homeless person will take your order and bring you your meal and coffee. It was great, but it took most of the day. When I had the money, I would pay for the meal. Most people paid to support the restaurant and keep it going. We have to beg to get money, but it is worth it to pay for the meal. I cannot appear to be homeless or I will not find a job, and my sales career here is over. Who is going to buy anything from a homeless man?

The people I meet at the shelters are mostly people who have given up on themselves. They have what I refer to as a jail mentality. They do not care how they look or how they dress and they use the foulest language they can think of. They have no problem talking about being in prison while on public transportation, or discussing beating their girlfriends and reporting to the Department of Corrections. They discuss all the meth that they smoked. They have lost any pride they ever had. I will never understand what brings someone to the point that he or she no longer cares about themselves. Bipolar people have a lot of pride. This is a trait found in most bipolar levels one to three, according to my psychiatrist. Because of my pride, I cannot allow myself to be like the others. I cannot relate to woman my own age. Because of this, I get along better with much younger people. I love young people and I love being around young people. They make me feel young. I have always taken care of myself and tried to look the best I could with what I had at the time. I did not know it, but later in life, this has helped me tremendously. Even now that I am homeless, I can still look good and people would never guess that I do not have a home. Because of my ability to act and be "on" almost all the time, I can convince people that I am a successful salesperson.

It is true that I am of above-average intelligence. Almost all bipolar persons have above-average intelligence. This is why we get into so much trouble. This is not a blessing, but instead actually hurts us. It is a curse. How many times I have wished that I was stupid or brain damaged rather than being bipolar! I have a very large suitcase full of clothes; the only possessions I have left of my life. I cannot take it when I go to look for work. I cannot appear to be homeless. Since I look nice and can talk well, I can go to any large hotel and they will check my bags for free.

My days consist of waking up, maybe at the airport, maybe outside, or under a bridge or in a doorway. I could not stay at the airport very long because the Portland police would throw me out. I would pick up my suitcase from whichever hotel I had left it at. I would take my suitcase to the Greyhound bus station and clean up the best that I could, if security did not throw me out. I would change my clothes and find another hotel where I would check my suitcase again, and then go look for work. The hotels began to know me, and I am sure they wondered what I was doing, but perhaps they knew and felt sorry for me.

I had to beg for money, or I would not have had any money at all. Sometimes I had to find a Laundromat so I could put my clothes in the dryer and remove the wrinkles, when I had the money. I could not wash my clothes most of the time, and had to wear the same clothes for a week.

I watched the other homeless people beg for money. They would say,

"You can't spare a quarter, could ya?" That was a double negative. Or, they would say, "You couldn't spare a cigarette, could ya?" I learned from them very fast. I would say, "Could you spare a fellow American a dollar?" I was amazed at how much money I could get that way. Not enough to live on, but I did get by. It paid for cigarettes and vodka. I had no meds for a while so I could not sleep at night, the vodka helped me sleep. There is nothing worse than lying under a bridge and not being able to sleep. It is horrible. I thought about how completely screwed up everything was.

MY BIPOLAR

I have researched my condition because I wanted to know what's wrong with me. It is important to know that when someone is bipolar, that person does not realize it. Everyone in the world can see it, but not the person who has it. I felt that I was normal and the whole world was wrong. Even after taking my meds for a long time, if I stopped the meds my ex, Delarosa, would know instantly. She would always ask me if I took my meds. She could see a difference in me that I did not see.

This is important, because you will ask why I did the things that I did. You will look for a logical answer, but there is none. Everyone who has had a relationship with someone who is bipolar will always blame the person who is bipolar. They will say the bipolar person set out to sabotage the relationship and the persons involved. They will also say that the bipolar person set out to deliberately harm them and the family. They will say that the bipolar condition can be an excuse for their actions. They will say that bipolar people are evil. Nothing could be further from the truth. I have firsthand knowledge of what people have told me; my former wife is an example. She will never believe that I did not set out to destroy her. She will never understand the bipolar condition. She hates me for what I have done to her. She has closed her mind to any reasonable explanation of what happened in our marriage.

It is for this reason that I wrote this book, to help people understand bipolar disorder. People are not ready to accept bipolar as a legitimate illness, in part because bipolar is new as a diagnosis for a mental condition. It may seem hard to believe that I could not control what I did, but it is true. I could no more control what I did than I could control the weather. People ask why I could not make the right choices. They will say that I knew right from wrong, and I chose the wrong way to go. They feel that I should pay for what I did. If someone is mentally retarded, people forgive him or her, and try to help them. If someone is schizophrenic, people feel sorry for them. If someone has a personality disorder, people look at him or her as crazy and try to help them. When someone has Alzheimer's, we take care of him or her. Not so with bipolar.

My mind raced all of my life, so fast I could not even think. I had no time for that; I was busy. I felt like I was going 100 mph all the time. Also, the only thing I could think about was my immediate needs or desires. I needed something risky, something that made me feel alive. I needed the thrill of danger and uncertainty in my life. I wanted to feel good all the time. It could be sex, gambling, drugs and alcohol, or the speed of racing cars. I never had time to make a sound decision. I never considered the penalties for my actions; I just did it. My life was hell; my own personal hell. This was especially true when I went into my depressive state. I hated it more than I could express here. When manic, I could talk almost anyone into almost anything, and I did this many times. Selling someone on an idea is simply transference of energy from one person to another. I had an abundance of energy. I am very spontaneous about everything in my life. Bipolar disorder. People are not ready to accept bipolar as a legitimate illness, in part because bipolar is new as a diagnosis for a mental condition. It may seem hard to believe that I could not control what I did, but it is true. I could no more control what I did than I could control the weather. People ask why I could not make the right choices. They will say that I knew right from wrong, and I chose the wrong way to go. They feel that I should pay for what I did. If someone is mentally retarded, people forgive him or her, and try to help them. If someone is schizophrenic, people feel sorry for them. If someone has a personality disorder, people look at him or her as crazy and try to help them. When someone has Alzheimer's, we take care of him or her. Not so with bipolar.

My mind raced all of my life, so fast I could not even think. I had no time for that; I was busy. I felt like I was going 100 mph all the time. Also, the only thing I could think about was my immediate needs or desires. I needed something risky, something that made me feel alive. I needed the thrill of danger and uncertainty in my life. I wanted to feel good all the time. It could be sex, gambling, drugs and alcohol, or the speed of racing cars. I never had time to make a sound decision. I never considered the penalties for my actions; I just did it. My life was hell; my own personal hell. This was especially true when I went into my depressive state. I hated it more than I could express here. When manic, I could talk almost anyone into almost anything, and I did this many times. Selling someone on an idea is simply transference of energy from one person to another. I had an abundance of energy. I am very spontaneous about everything in my life.

How many times have I heard people say, "Oh, just take your meds and you will be fine"? How little they really know what hell bipolar is. Hell on earth. Yes, a living hell that destroys lives. Yes. The hell I lived all of my life, and I did not know what to do or that I even had a problem until I was fifty eight years old. My brain flashes from moment to moment. Ideas and thoughts flash by much faster than other people's. It is very hard to concentrate on any one thing long enough to complete anything. Bipolar people often start many different projects without completing any of them.

The only way that I can write this book is because of the medication that I take every day. There are drugs that a bipolar person can take to help them live a better life. It takes many attempts to find the right combination that works for the individual. This could easily take over a year. Only a psychiatrist can prescribe these medications.

It takes many sessions to begin to form an opinion on what drugs will work and then proceed from there. For me, I started on lithium, as most psychiatrists would prescribe. That was to control my manic state. I could not take the lithium very long because of my liver and the hepatitis C that I have, but it did work. For depression, I took Welbutrin, very large doses at first, nine hundred milligrams. For my sleep problem, I took Seroquel, three hundred milligrams to start. Seroquel can also be an antipsychotic drug.

I can only say that Seroquel is a miracle drug. For the first time that I can remember, I slept a full eight hours and I felt great when I woke up. Seroquel is not habit forming. It is not an opiate or narcotic of any kind, but it works incredibly well. The only problem is the price. A one hundred milligram tablet costs six dollars, and I had to take three. That was eighteen dollars a day just for that. Along with the other medication, the total was thirty-five dollars every day of my life. In addition, the psychiatric treatment was one hundred dollars an hour. It is easy to see that I needed medical insurance. Of course, I did not have it, so the state had to pay.

My psychiatrist started me on an antipsychotic drug called Neurontin to slow the firing of my brain. It worked well, but I could not live a normal life or operate a car or anything else. I called this drug a frontal lobotomy pill, because that is how I felt. I was taking eighteen hundred milligrams at first. I was nonfunctional. This trial and error method lasted over a year. I never blamed my psychiatrist for this. She was wonderful and I loved her. She helped me out tremendously. She took me through many dark areas that I had locked away. In addition, she helped me with my bipolar.

I decided to write this book so that others may have an understanding of the dark side of bipolar disorder; in the hope that I can help just one person who may be suffering from this hideous disease. I wrote this book for anyone who may read it and say, "Hey! That sounds like me, or someone I know!", and then seek help and treatment.

The truth that I have written in this book may scare and confuse you. It might make you sad, and maybe cry. It could, at times, make you laugh. However, make no mistake; the truth is very frightening and may disturb a lot of you. I chose not to hide the facts, but to bring them out so everyone could read them, no matter how painful or embarrassing this would be for me. You, the reader, deserve to know the truth about me and my battle with bipolar disorder; a disease that knows no logic, and beyond what most people can understand. What you need to know is that bipolar is the only mental illness that can be completely controlled by medication. You are born with bipolar. It is hereditary. You cannot catch it like a virus. There is no cure for bipolar disorder, but it can be controlled with medications.

The truth about my story is I am one of many thousands of people who suffer from this illness. Many are misdiagnosed or not diagnosed at all. It is important to note that I am not a psychiatrist, or a doctor of any kind. I am simply attempting to explain my life with bipolar disorder. The details of my life are very important to show that there are many factors that can mask a bipolar diagnosis. The bipolar condition only gets worse with time, and never gets better on its own. Over many years, I can tell you that it definitely gets worse. I am living proof of that.

I left out many of the dates in this story, mainly because I cannot remember them. The actual dates are not that important for this book. One very important thing to mention here is that I never tried to hide what I did behind bipolar. I have to take full responsibility for my actions, and I have. I have paid for what I've done in many ways. We all have our own private hell. One way or another, we all pay for what we do in life.

My price was extremely high. It was a waste of a lifetime. If I sound severe, put yourself in my place at sixty-two years old. **Life is a drawing without an eraser!** God, I wish I had known that earlier. I wish I were not bipolar. I have cried a thousand times writing this book.

November, 1953

I was seven years old then. That is as far back as I can remember. We lived in Brooklyn, New York, in a tenement building (brownstone) with thirty other families. We lived in what they called cold water flat, which was a single floor apartment without hot water. My grandmother, Leona; grandfather, Charles; my two brothers, Mike and Joel; and I lived there.

We were raised Roman Catholic. Joel and I grew up as strict Catholics. Catholicism had me afraid of Jesus and of God. We believed that we were going to burn in hell no matter what we did. There was no reason for us to be good or to do right the thing. There was no reason at all. I could not understand why God could be so mean. It did not make any sense. If he is a loving caring God, then why does he hate us so much? Why are we going to hell? There was no reason to pray. It would not matter anyway. In addition, we had monsters for parents. They would sin all week long, and then go to church, and everything was okay. They were both street angels and house devils. They had both of us totally screwed up over religion. We had hypocrites for parents. Of course, we blamed ourselves for that. We felt we must deserve hell anyway. It took a lifetime to realize the truth. How cruel can anyone be to do this to young children? I will not go into a lot of detail about the people involved in my story.

This is not a novel and all that detail would confuse the reader and take away from the real meaning of this book. Our grandparents (who later became our parents through adoption) raised my brothers Mike, Joel and I. Mike was one year older than I was, and I was one year older than Joel. Our birth mother, Francis, was an extremely beautiful girl and became involved with older men at a very young age. Francis became involved with the Italians in Brooklyn. Three different men knocked her up then left her.

I remember the age of seven because, at that time, New York State had a law that stated children in our situation couldn't be legally adopted until they went before a judge and said that they wanted to live with the people that would adopt them. For that, you had to be at least seven years old. I was afraid of my grandparents and they threatened all three of us.

Our grandparents told us to say yes to the judge and we did. At that time, we lived one block from a bar called Eddie's. Leona spent most of her time there. She would often have to be helped home because of her drunkenness. Our grandfather joined the Merchant Marines, and then we were alone with Leona. When he did come home from over there, all he did was beat us anyway. He made fun of us all the time. He called me "egghead" because I loved eggs. He would always tell me how ugly and worthless I was. I grew up thinking that I was ugly. It took many years to figure out he was wrong. My brothers and I often went hungry. We had to steal food to eat. Nickel for snacks. It did not take us long before we learned to steal food, and only the best.

The Italian families gave us work, selling drugs for them. Because we were kids, when we did get busted, we went to a juvenile home instead of jail, and that was better than our home anyway. The Italians never really gave us much money, but it seemed like a lot to us at the time. Heroin was popular then. We delivered a lot of it, mostly to blacks. The Italians hated blacks. As we grew older, we realized that we could make a lot more money selling the heroin ourselves. We bought the heroin from other Italian families for less money, and then sold it for a higher profit. When Mike was arrested for selling drugs, all of our drug sales ended. When the Italians in our neighborhood found out what happened, they slapped the shit out of us. They always slapped our faces and that hurt like hell. Then, we had to sell the drugs for free until we paid back our debt.

I really hated all the movies about the Italian mobs. They always glamorized them. In reality, they were cold, heartless people. They never really had anything except clothes and shoes. Some had cars. Other than that, they were like everyone else trying to survive. Mike was gone for three months and we had no contact with him. mike eventually went to live with our mother, Francis. That was a big mistake, as you will see later.

Charles joined the Merchant Marines because he was hiding from someone. We did not know who or why. When Charles left the Merchant Marines, we moved twenty-six times in one year; not just different addresses, but different towns and cities. Men would come to our house and ask for him. Some wore suits and ties. They threatened us if we didn't tell them where he was, but we never did. Charles once hid under the floorboards in the kitchen. He dug a crawl space under the floor where he could hide. As I look back now, he was probably hiding from the mafia. No one ever figured out why. He died with that secret. Charles and Leona fought constantly when he was home.

Friends and school were a big problem because we moved around so much. We only had each other: my brother Joel and me. Mike was not around for us. One of our moves ended us in Fairbanks, Alaska. Joel and I grew up there as far as life outside of New York. Charles, Jr lived in Fairbanks at the time and talked Charles and Leona into moving there. We witnessed a lot of physical violence between our grandparents. Once we were eating dinner, and they were fighting, as usual. Leona picked up a two-pronged fork and stuck that right into Charles's chest. There was blood everywhere. Charles had to pull the fork out of his chest. He then dislocated her shoulder and threw her to the floor. We called the police. The police took them to the hospital.

ALASKA

May 1959

On the way to Alaska, they started to fight again. Leona clutched her purse, and then hit Charles in the face with it. We were going about fifty miles an hour. She had knocked his glasses off and Charles could not see anything. There was snow on the road, and we started to swerve back and forth across the road. Joel and I were scared and thought we might die. We were screaming for them to stop. The Alcan Highway is raised three feet above the ground to keep the road from flooding. The car left the road on the left side, and then crashed into some trees. We had to wait for a truck to come by to pull the car back on the road. Luckily, no one was hurt physically, but we were mentally.

When we stopped for gas and to get something to eat, Leona had to use the toilet and so did Charles. She went first, and then Charles followed. After a while, Charles came back. We asked where Leona was, and Charles said he did not know. Joel and I went to look for her. She was lying on the floor at the bottom of the stairs. She said Charles threw her down the stairs. She had a dislocated shoulder. Charles and the owner of the gas stop put her shoulder back in place, and sat her down at a table. We ate and left, and Leona never said much after that all the way to Alaska.

I remember the crazy things we did there which almost ended our lives several times. I will refer to Charles and Leona as my parents because through adoption they were the only parents that we knew. Charles, Jr., gave both Joel and I twenty-two caliber rifles. We thought we were big hunters. We went off into the woods to hunt game with a twenty- two rifle. We found some tracks in the snow and followed them. We did not know what kind of animal left the tracks, but it looked like a dog or large cat. We must have followed the tracks for a mile. We were not dressed for the weather, and we soon had snow in our shoes. Our fingers were cold and freezing. We did not even have decent hats. Up ahead, we heard what sounded like a baby crying. We looked at each other, and then Joel said, "What was that?" I said, "What would a baby be doing out here?" Just ahead, we could see a cabin. The door was partially opened and the tracks led right into the cabin. As we approached the cabin, we heard the crying again, only much louder. The cries seemed to come from the inside the cabin. Joel said, "That is no baby!", and I agreed. Joel entered the cabin first and cocked the twenty-two rifle. I was just behind him and cocked my gun.

The cabin was a single room with a stove in the middle. There was no heat and no one there. It looked like the place had been ransacked. There was empty food containers scattered all over the place. At the back of the room was a hole in the floor, like a cellar. We both approached the cellar, and then I looked down into the hole. To our surprise, there was a large cat down there, with babies. Before we could move, the cat screamed, and then jumped at us. The cat was a big lynx, but we did not realize that. We also did not realize that she was protecting her young. We both froze. I remembered that I felt paralyzed. I was so scared that I could not move at all.

This seemed to last a long time; I don't know how long it was. Finally, Joel said, "Let's get the hell out of here!", and then we both jumped up and ran like hell. Joel left his gun by the cellar door. I could not let go of mine. It was clamped in my hand and I could not let go of it. We ran almost all the way back home. Later, Charles Jr. told us the cat was a lynx, and we were damn lucky the lynx did not come after us. It was several days before Charles Jr. went back for the gun, but only when he saw the cat leave using binoculars. Joel and I never went near the cabin again.

Another time, we were out in the woods with Charles Jr. and we had no guns. We were headed for the Tanana River where we could fish. It was spring, and the ice on the river had broken up from the winter. We set up by the shore of the river and then started baiting the hooks. We could see the fish in the water, and they were big. It was exciting for Joel and me, having come from Brooklyn. As we baited our hooks, we heard a loud roar behind us. We all looked back and saw a brown bear standing there looking at us. He was a couple hundred feet from us, and he was just looking at us as he paced back and forth. He looked like he was six feet tall, and had big teeth and enormous claws. I froze and could not move. I was paralyzed once more.

Charles Jr. was trying to figure a way out for us, but we did not have anywhere to go. We were against the river and had two choices: run into the river or run along the river. Either way, the bear would get us. The river was so cold that we would have died in ten minutes, and the bear would come after us anyway. Charles Jr. told us not to move, so we all froze right there. In what seemed to be a lifetime, the bear started to move away, but he was still pacing back and forth while watching us and he roared. I can truly say that I pissed my pants and could not do anything about it. The bear moved away far enough so we could very slowly walk along the river. Soon he left, and we were definitely scared. We grabbed our fishing equipment and left. We never went anywhere again without a gun, and a big gun, not a twenty-two.

Then there was the propane tank incident. Our father was working out of town. He worked on the DEW line (distant early warning system) and had left us with Leona. We cooked with propane, and when we ran out Joel and I would hitchhike to the town of North Pole to fill the propane tank, then hitchhike back home again. Back then, hitchhiking was very easy because most of the vehicles on the road were military, and they always stopped for us.

I watched Charles Jr. hook up the propane tank many times, so I knew how to do that. After the tank was connected, Charles Jr. would light a match and place the flame near the connection. If there was a leak, he would tighten the connection until the flame went out. That way, there was never a leak with the tank. The propane tank connected to a pipe outside the house. I connected the tank, tightened the fitting and lit the match. There was a tiny leak, so I let it burn as I tightened the connection. The valve on the propane tank broke off, and the flames shot up about the height of the house. At first, we ran like hell, and then we realized it was just a flame. What we did not know is that when all the pressure left the tank the flame would go inside the tank and cause an explosion. That was exactly what happened. The tank exploded, putting a big hole in the side of the house.

The force of that explosion blew us both off our feet and about twenty feet from the tank on our backs. There was an army jeep going by the house when the tank blew. The two soldiers had seen the smoke and heard the explosion. They brought us to the hospital. Leona was fine. There was no fire, because the blast must have blown the flames out. We were very lucky. All we had were burns. Our hair was burnt along with our eyebrows. We were sore for a couple of days, but other than that, we survived.

I stole the family car that was sitting in our driveway. Charles was on the DEW line at the time and we were left with Leona. I figured it was a good idea. Leona was drunk, so Joel and I went for a ride.

I decided to take the car on the tank trail. The army tanks cannot drive on the road because they would destroy it. The tanks have their own roads called "tank trails". I did not realize how bad the tank trails were. There were holes twelve feet deep and they had a lot of water in them. I drove into one of these holes. We were hopelessly stuck. The top of the car was far below the ground. We climbed out of the hole and looked at the car. There was no way we could get the car out. We both sat there looking at the car for hours. I was not going to go home without the car.

We heard the sounds of tanks in the distance. I figured we were screwed for sure. Within thirty minutes, we saw the tanks approaching. Three tanks pulled up and then stopped. We did not have to say a word. They knew what had happened. One tank stopped while the other two continued around the hole in the trail. The young man said, "Looks like you need some help." I said yes. The man hooked a long chain to the frame of the car and then to the tank. Effortlessly, the tank backed up and slowly pulled the car out. He said, "Maybe you should take the car home now." I agreed, and he left.

I drove the car back to the road, and then we went home. The car was covered with mud. The floor was soaked from the water. We spent hours cleaning it. Leona never realized what we had done. When Charles came home and looked at the car, he knew something had happened. He asked us about it and we both said we did not have a clue.

We tried to enroll in school, but when we were tested, we were two grades behind the other kids our age. After testing us again, they put us only one grade behind. I struggled because I was totally lost in math. I had a big problem concentrating in school. My mind drifted and I could not control it. My mind was everywhere except in school. I could not follow the teacher at all. I was lost. This must have seemed serious to my teacher because she sent me to the principal, who called Leona and told her about the problem. The principal suggested that I go to a doctor.

We could not afford a doctor so I went to the county hospital. The doctor there diagnosed me as hyperactive with ADD. He prescribed Ritalin. Ritalin is a speed pill, which actually has the opposite effect on hyperactive people. Back then, the medical community did not know enough about bipolar disorder to make a diagnosis. They often diagnosed bipolar as schizophrenia or a personality disorder. I must have fit in there somewhere.

I will explain the personality disorder. When information comes in to our brain, we process this information and then act on that information. A person who has a personality disorder will process this information very differently. What comes out is so bizarre; no one can understand them or what they did. This information seems very real for people with this disorder. However, it is actually extremely harmful to anyone they meet.

I always had a lot of trouble sleeping. I would go to bed at 9:00-11:00 pm; it did not matter what time I went to bed. I would wake up a couple of hours later and then stay awake the rest of the night. I did this for weeks and never got tired. My brain would tell my body that it was not tired. I could not understand why everyone else slept so much. I could do so much more than they could because I never slept very much. I made fun of anyone who slept more than a couple hours, including my family. Mike and Joel never had this problem and they never understood me. Leona was so screwed up that it was hard to tell what was wrong with her, but she was alcoholic and also took many prescribed meds on top of that. (I will share more about her later).

The manic feeling I had without my meds was incredible. I remember how much I enjoyed the feeling. I could do anything, and I did, many times. I began to skip school and hang out with people much older than me. They dropped out of school, smoked, drank and chased women. I felt like I belonged with them. Now that I look back, I was a risk taker, as most bipolar people are. One of the places we lived was Watertown, New York. It was a farm community, and Joel and I hated it. We were not farmers. We were city boys. Our neighbor rented us the house that we lived in. We could not believe that we had an outhouse and a manual water pump in the front yard. We were going to run away, so we started our plan.

In the meantime, we worked on the turkey farm that our neighbor owned. We worked all summer collecting turkey eggs. At the end of the summer, we were paid thirteen dollars each, which Leona took. I wanted a fishing pole and after working all summer long, I did not get it.

We had many apple trees on the property. Joel and I had apple fights all the time. We built forts out of junk lumber. I can tell you that it hurts to be hit with apples, especially when hit with the small unripe apples. We were bruised all over our bodies from apples. We eventually moved back to New York.

BACK TO NEW YORK

October, 1962

Sammy, one of my best friends, was a tall, good-looking Italian boy who was five years older than me. Sammy showed me how to approach girls and older women. I loved it, especially since I felt ugly as a child anyway. I met Sammy in Brooklyn, which is where we wound up, again, after Alaska. Sammy and I would take a Greyhound bus from New York to Miami Beach, Florida. There, we hung out at the Fountain Blue Hotel where older women would pick us up. The women had money lots of money. They were married and always alone. These women would take us out to lunch, buy us drinks, and treat us like kings. They would buy us clothes, shoes and give us money.

The drinking age was eighteen at that time. I had false identification. They would get us drunk, and all we had to do was spend the night with them, and of course have sex with them. I did not know it then, but they were actually sex abusers. They paid us so they could carry out their sexual fantasies with young boys. In the morning, Sammy and I would meet at the restaurant and talk about the night before. We\ would joke about being whores, but that was fine with me. Some of the women were good looking. Soon after I met Sammy, I dropped out of school completely and stopped taking my meds. I loved the feeling of being manic, although at the time I did not know what manic was. I knew I did not like the Ritalin.

I had friends in Brooklyn from childhood. We always caught up with each other. Everyone had their own little business going on. Sammy was very good at passing bad checks. Pauli was good at credit cards. Back then, there were no computers and it took a week or so for the bad checks and credit cards to show up. It was easy money. I sold drugs and made good money. Frankie, well, he was good at stealing from train cars and delivery trucks. He would pay off the truck drivers, and then they would let him steal the trucks. They would report to the police that some tall black man took their truck.

We always spent everything we made. We had to keep up the appearance of being well-to-do. It was all very crazy, but that was reality for us. Sammy and I broke into a train car, and it was full of cookies, all different kinds of cookies. There must have been a couple hundred cases. All of Brooklyn had cookies. We sold what we could and then gave away the rest. We all had to pay the Italian families a part of everything we made. In return, we avoided being busted. It was worth the money Eventually everyone was busted anyway and most were facing federal time. That is when everyone ratted everyone else out. If you were facing thirty-five years in prison, what would you do? My drug sales were federal because I crossed state lines into

Jersey. Of course, you know the rest. Everyone went into witness protection programs and gave up their families. Believe me; it was not fun when I had to testify in front of the people being prosecuted. The chances of living were not very good, and we knew that.

The strange thing about this was we all wound up in San Jose, California, and we all knew each other. This did not make any sense. Maybe they thought we would kill each other off. The FBI who kept track of us were called handlers. We all had the same handler there. They always checked on us. Even stranger than that, eventually we all wound up in Spokane, Washington.

LOS ANGELES
November, 1963

I met a person named Frank. Again, he was older than I was by six years. Frank was from L.A. He told me all about California and the way people lived there. I never believed him. We used to look through Time-Life magazine and see the ranch style homes with swimming pools and two car garages, but I never believed them. I thought all of that crap about the lifestyle in California was just for movie stars. I never told anyone where I was going because of witness protection. We arrived in L.A. four months before we went to San Jose. It was like being born again. I could not believe my eyes. I wished everyone in New York could see through my eyes what I was seeing. It was all true; the magazines and Frank. They were right.

This was paradise. Frank took me to Santa Monica pier and we spent three days there. We went to Long Beach and it was incredible. It was late fall then and the temperature was in the 80's. We had federal money to take care of ourselves. Frank introduced me to Steve Galliano, who owned a pizza restaurant and he took me in as if I was his own son. Frank was killed in a motorcycle accident shortly after that.

Steve taught me how to cook Italian, and actually run his restaurant for him. Steve taught me everything I needed to know about managing a restaurant. He set me up with a room in downtown L.A. Steve trusted me, and he could take time off and not worry about his business. He actually took a week off, went to Italy, and left me in charge.

I guess being manic helped me a lot at the time. I was a very quick learner and never needed very much sleep. I never took anything from Steve. I had a lot of respect for him. He was the father I never had.

Soon I bought a car. It was a Corvair Monza. It was a bright red convertible with wire wheels. I loved that car. I only had the car a month, and then blew the engine. It was air-cooled and the fan belt broke on the freeway. The sun was bright and shining on the dash and I didn't see the warning light. I bought the car from Tony, a friend of Steve's. He was about seven years older than me, and he taught me a lot.

Tony was trying to get into the movies. He wanted to be an actor more than anything else in the world, like everyone else in Los Angeles. Tony had taken voice lessons, so he could project his voice. Tony was a good-looking man. He talked me into signing up with the screen actor's guild as an extra. I actually played a dead army soldier in Rat Patrol. They paid us twenty-five dollars a day. They never showed our faces; otherwise they would have to pay us a lot more. Rat Patrol was a television show at that time. I drove everyone crazy trying to get into movies so I could act. I realized that I had been acting all my life. I just called it "being on". The acting bug had me.

I quit working for Steve, and then had to go to San Jose. I had money, but took a job in sales, selling Kirby Vacuum cleaners. What attracted me to that position was the ad. "Travel the West Coast!" and "Sell with the Best!" What I really liked was the travel, and the fact that we would travel in groups of fifteen. The groups were co-ed. All I could think about was party time.

I was very good at selling the vacuums. I sold two out of three demos. I was making, on average, six hundred dollars a week. It was easy. The Kirby sold itself on the demos. The big thing was vacuuming the bottom of the mattress where their feet would be. The demo used a special adapter, not a bag. This adapter used a small white pad where the vacuum bag would be. When we vacuumed the bed, the pad would fill up with grey ash about an inch deep, which was dead skin. The people freaked out, and then they would buy the vacuum. We never told them this was perfectly normal, and that every mattress had the same ash.

Some of my other sales were for cookware, encyclopedias, magazines and Bibles. Whatever I sold, I was very good at it. I could out-think people, and I was going so fast with so much energy that people did not have a chance to say "no". I followed a salesman named Zig Ziggler, who was named the best salesman of the year for many years. Zig sold many of the same products that I sold. Every time I could, I would read about him and listen to what he said at sales conventions.

The downside of being "on" was being "off"; the depression part of bipolar condition. When I cycled to the depressive side, I would hide in my room, watch TV, and not talk to anyone at all. I would miss work and everything else in the world. I would cry and became very sad. All I could do was escape into the television.

I am very lucky because my depression lasted only two to three days. It could have been much worse. The doctors told me there are eleven different levels of the disease. I am bipolar one. My cycle runs mostly in the manic stage with a short cycle in the depressive side. Some bipolar people are the opposite; they are depressed most of the time.

Being manic is one of the greatest feelings. It is like being in a plane at 35,000 feet. The depressive side is like jumping out of that plane. I wondered many times how far down I could go. When I look back at my life, it looks like a nuclear explosion happened right in the middle of my life.

I remember blaming objects for my problems. I never had any patience at all, and if something did not work correctly, I would destroy the object itself. I would blame inanimate objects for my lack of patience. This self-destructive temper has lasted throughout my life.

WOODSTOCK

The sixties were here.

I remember the Beatles on the Ed Sullivan Show. From that point on, I was never the same. The sixties were the very best time of my entire life. I found drugs: grass, acid, cocaine, mushrooms and anything else I could get my hands on. Free love was upon us and all I had to do was ask a woman if she wanted to ball, and that was that. We got high and balled all day and night.

I was never happier; I fit right in and all my problems went away. I was good looking, smart, loved to party, and I took acid almost every day, it seemed. I tried other boys and they were fun. I laughed all the time. I had friends, many friends.

I sold acid to pay for the acid I took along with the grass we smoked. I always had a sheet of 100 hits of acid called a "windowpane" or "orange sunshine", "purple haze". The acid we had was LSD 25; the most potent LSD you could get from Berkeley, California. Sugar cubes were also popular because one tiny drop on a sugar cube is all anyone ever needed. Most of this LSD was made by Timothy Leary at the UC Berkley Campus. He was a highly influential American psychologist and writer, known in particular for advocating the therapeutic benefits of psychedelic drugs. A hugely controversial figure during the 1960s and 1970s, he defended the use of the drug LSD. Everyone had a nickname and mine was "Rabbit". Everyone knew me as "Rabbit". During the late sixties, I traveled from Seattle to San Francisco and Berkeley then back again. My friends and I spent a lot of time in the Haight Asbury district of San Francisco. I had long hair and dirty, ragged jeans and tie-dyed shirts. I met Jimmy Hendricks in person at a concert in Seattle. We smoked some grass with him and talked. He seemed so young to play music like he did and he was one of us. He was twenty or twenty-one at that time.

I also met Janis Joplin. My girlfriend at the time was in the women's room with her. She and Janis came out laughing; they had been snorting coke. Janis had a large drink and seemed really stoned, but so were we. Janis always had a drink in her hand. God bless her little soul. We partied for a bit, and then she went on stage and sang the blues. Back then, it was easy to meet the entertainers. Like the Grateful Dead who played in a bar called the Bodega. The bar capacity was only about ninety people.

My brother, Joel, was still in New York. He had gone to jail for selling drugs. I stayed in touch with him. When Joel got out, he told me about Woodstock. I heard stories about a great big concert in New York, but I really did not know much about it. I had a girlfriend at the time (Rosie) and I had an old Bonneville station wagon, so we loaded up the car with all our belongings. We put paisley curtains in the back and side windows. Off we went to New York and Woodstock. By that time, my manic side was crazy, and I did many risky things, like shooting up drugs; mostly meth. Back then meth was clean. They used ether as a base. One shot would keep you up twenty-fours, easy. I made some very bad decisions then without thinking about the outcome. Rosie was a very wild girl, and now that I look back, she may have been bipolar.

On that trip to New York, we did not plan anything. We did not have enough money to make the trip, and did not count on anything going wrong with the car. In some strange, little town in Texas, the car broke down. At that time, Texas was very red neck. They did not like hippies and they did not like us.

We had to sell some things to get money to fix the car. We took our camera to a pawnshop to sell it. While we waited for the clerk to go get the money from the back room, he called the police. The police did not like us at all. We had no receipt for the camera, so they arrested us and charged us with vagrancy.

We had to call people in San Francisco to wire us money so we could pay our fines. Oddly enough, our fines were not set until the police knew how much money we could get from back home. Even stranger than that, the fines were exactly the amount that we had wired to us from home. We had to wire for more money to get the hell out of there.

While we were waiting for the second wire to come, they let us out of jail. Rosie thought it might be a good idea to walk up and down the sidewalks singing profane language repeatedly. Everyone was freaking out as they watched us walk down the street; bad idea. So here are the police again. By that time, we found out the car was fixed, and we got the money, paid the bill and we split. The police followed us until we were out of town.

We met some wonderful people on that trip and partied all the way to New York. It was like a week and a half before we arrived in New York State. Joel had moved to upstate New York by then, so that is where we went: Rochester.

When people say; if you remember the sixties you were not there, they are telling the truth. All I remember is the love everyone had, the drugs and the incredible entertainment through the sixties and seventies. By the time we met Joel and finally made Woodstock, it was already way out of control. The fences were plowed down by the people. There was no one to take tickets anymore, and it seemed like everyone in the country was there. It was overwhelming, and looked like the coming of Christ where everyone wanted to see Him. I remember a Grateful Dead concert we had gone to. It was in Watkins Glenn, New York at the speedway. There were about two hundred thousand people there. It was the second largest concert next to Woodstock.

The one thing I remember about Woodstock is you could never see what was going on anywhere but in your immediate area. Wondering around to find someone while stoned on acid was almost impossible and it seemed to take all day. We climbed the speaker towers to look for people. The manic side made it easier for me. I always had a lot of energy no matter what drug I took. The music was incredible and the sound systems were very loud and powerful. Then the rain came. The rain never really seemed to stop the parties. No one much cared after a while anyway.

I tried heroin but it never worked for me. I never got a rush from heroin. I would smoke grass and get a burst of energy; jump in the car and off we'd go. Everyone else seemed to be laid back while I went like hell. When I first started to smoke grass, I would make fun of all the California people who would just sit and veg out. They would get munchies, eat and just sit and trip out on the music. I did not understand that at all.

I had arrived! My life was good, in fact better than it ever was. As the sixties rolled on, though, everything seemed to change. The free love seemed to leave us, and in its place came people who were only trying to rip everyone off. It had become a time when you could not trust anyone. My brain did not want to let go of that time; I held on to it for dear life. However, it changed anyway; I guess it had to end. The drug scene changed from peaceful, loving people to everyone out for themselves. My manic side helped a lot then; I could out think most people and that kept me from being ripped off most of the time. The drug scene changed to more hard-core drugs: cocaine, heroin, hashish and opium. There were still times of fun and laughter drinking and smoking grass, but it was different. Charles Manson was in the headlines and cults were popping up everywhere.

We traveled a lot then from the east coast to the west and Alaska. I remember Fillmore West and Fillmore East, as they had the biggest and best concerts. I lived like a gypsy for years. I stayed in touch with Joel through all this. Mike was not involved with the sixties or with us. He went to live with Francis, and that was the worst thing he could have done. Whenever I saw him or heard about Mike, he was on tranquilizers and had become a nervous wreck. Mike had a mental breakdown and was in a mental hospital in upstate New York. Francis had treated him terribly, as we later found out. Mike apparently jumped from the fifth floor window of the hospital and died. I never believed that, and neither did anyone else. We all thought he was pushed from the window. Mike was too much of a man to do that. He was always a macho man. He lifted weights and had an incredible build. When I did confront Francis I went crazy on her and my true manic side came out. I made her realize what she had done to us and how we paid for what she did. Then she blamed Mike for the nervous breakdown that he had. I have never seen her since that time. She died. I never forgave her.

Leona and Charles had other children besides Francis: Charles Jr. and David, Loretta and Eleanor. They became our half brothers and sisters although we never saw much of them when we were growing up. Once they left the hell of being brought up by Charles and Leona, they never came back, not even to help us. David married and died from alcoholism. Eleanor married an alcoholic and he died very young. Charles Jr. married twice and had four children. He is still alive today at eighty-two years old. He now has Alzheimer's disease. Loretta married a lawyer who defended the mafia. He was pushed in front of a subway train. He died instantly when his body hit the third rail before the train came. Loretta is still alive. She is eighty-three now. Leona wound up in a mental hospital three times for drinking and taking powerful pain meds.

To understand what our childhood was like you first have to know Leona. Leona was an immigrant from Poland. She came through Ellis Island in New York where she met Charles. She no doubt had a hard if not horrible life herself. She was a total alcoholic. The things she did to us were pure horror.

Imagine if you will a child lying in bed maybe seven or eight years old. The child wakes up and something is wrong it is hard to breath; there is smoke everywhere. The child jumps out of bed and runs for the kitchen where the smoke is coming from. The child screams and no one wakes up. The child runs to wake his brother. They both run to the mother's room screaming, "Help! There's a fire! Mom, wake up! There's a fire in the kitchen!" However, mom never wakes up. Now imagine the children running back to the kitchen to put out the fire. They grab pots and pans and fill them with water to pour on the fire. The children run to the bedroom, pull the blankets from their bed, and lay them over the flames. They pour more and more water over the blankets. Soon the fire dies down and finally goes out. The fire department never came because, at that time, we moved to a very small town in upstate New York, and no one called the fire department. Back then, there was no 911 to call. Now imagine the children knew what really happened, they knew how the fire started. In fact, it was not the first time this had happened. We knew Leona had started the fire on purpose, as she had before. She would start the fire, go to bed, and pass out. Imagine how we felt when we went to bed and how hard it was to fall asleep

This was our childhood and the old man was gone, as usual. This was not the first time, and we knew it would not be the last. Leona would turn on the gas from the stove and go to sleep. She would build a fire under the car engine and pass out in bed. At times, we would find her passed out with her head in the oven with the gas turned on. As you can imagine, all that made us very insecure, and the one person we had to count on was doing it all herself.

I know what you thinking now. No wonder I grew up so screwed up and why I am bipolar. Although part of that is true, I am all screwed up; however, being bipolar ran in our family, as you can see, along with severe mental illness that was never diagnosed. Leona wound up in a mental hospital three times and she would sign herself in and out. The last time I remember her being in a mental hospital was when Charles signed her in. When someone commits you into a mental hospital, you cannot sign yourself out. The only way to get out is have the doctor release you. After a time, they would let her out again.

During all this, we were watched by babysitters paid for by the state. For the most part, they were terrible people; usually big, fat women that were dirty and smelled. We hated them and the garbage they fed us.

We would just steal food and eat that instead of their food. When I was about ten years old, we had a babysitter named Donna. Donna was about sixteen. She often played with herself in front of us. I loved to watch her and she even let me help. I had sex with her. It was great and it was my first time. I considered myself the weakest of the three of us. In fact, right now, writing this book is the most difficult task that I have ever taken on. All these feelings are surging to the surface again. Feelings I had put so far away that I thought I'd never remember or feel them ever again. I've cried all through this book. I mentioned this to my psychiatrist. A psychiatrist is the only type of doctor that can diagnose and prescribe medicine for bipolar. No other doctors can prescribe these meds, not even a psychologist. The feelings I have at this very moment are the feelings my psychiatrist has been trying to get me to feel for years now.

I grew up with a hatred for women, even though I had many lovers. I never trusted a woman for many years. I always knew they would hurt me. Someone brought that to my attention once, and I had never realized it until that moment. I had a very bad attitude towards women. My brother, Joel, died of a massive heart attack at the age of 46. Sometimes I miss Joel so much that I feel that I cannot go on without him, and I cry.

ADRIANE CORDAY

May 1970

I had my girlfriend, Rosie, who I had incredible times with. We partied together for what seemed years. We loved each other, and knew each other very well. Rosie was three years younger than I was. We took a lot of acid, smoked a lot grass and had incredible times. This was in San Jose, California. We got high on acid and had sex for eight hours at a time. When anyone is stoned on acid, time is irrelevant. Hours go by as minutes or a minute could last for hours. Therefore, to have sex for eight consecutive hours was common.

I remember I had three people in my car and we were all stoned. I waited for a stop sign to turn green. None of us realized that, and we stayed there for hours. Driving while stoned was not easy to do and it made me drive very carefully.

We spent many nights on the beach in Santa Cruz, stoned on acid, having sex and enjoying life, and we were not alone. We lived in a house just behind her mom's house. As her mom owned both, we did not pay any rent, so we had time and money to party. I sold acid and grass so we had money.

I have to explain something here. Charles told me one day that if you want to see what a woman looks like when she gets older, just look at her mother. Rosie's mom was way overweight with short hair and sack dresses. That scared me, because Rosie was a little heavy at the time. In retrospect that came true for Rosie. I saw her a couple years later in a store, and she look exactly like her mother, Charles was right, and I was sorry for Rosie.

I guess my time with Rosie was over because when I met Adriane everything changed. The truth is that I never thought I, Dominick Delarosso, could ever be with anyone like Adriane. She was from a middle class family. She was very responsible and very beautiful. She was seventeen at the time, and I was twenty-one. She had her own car and had a job. It is important to tell you that I always worked. I always had some kind of job and I always made money. The difference was that I was not responsible at all. Another trait of someone who may be bipolar is the recklessness of their lives, the irresponsibility they show, the lifestyle they live, and the decisions they make. When I met Adriane, I fell in love with her. Yes, it was love at first sight. I hurt Rosie a lot when I told her about Adriane, but I could not help it. I did not want to hurt her but I had to leave.

Adriane and I married shortly after that in Lake Tahoe. We lived for a time in the Santa Cruz Mountains. At that time, the sixties were slowing down, but there was still a lot going on and exciting things happening. It was the time of wife-swapping, and that is what we did. We attended parties for swinging partners. At some of these parties, when you arrived at the door the men would put their keys in a basket. The woman put their keys in another basket. Each woman or man would pick a key from the basket of the other sex, and that is who you had sex with. I found out that Adrian liked girls, also. That was okay. That made for some wild parties that would last all night.

Again being bipolar and a high-risk taker, I loved this idea as many people did. I know now that Adriane did not enjoy it as much as I did. I think she experimented with the idea, but did not enjoy it as much. This continued off and on through our relationship. We both found work and started our lives. But we could not make any decent money in California at that time. Joel was in Joel worked at Eastman Kodak Company and made good money there. Adriane and I applied Rochester, New York. We decided to move there to get work, and we did. for jobs, and we both were hired on. This time in our lives was bar party time. I never really partied with Joel in the bar scene. The drinking age then was eighteen, so we could all go to the bars together. It was incredible! Adriane and I made great money. We had great times together. We bought a new MGB and had a great life. However, there was a lot of irresponsibility with both of us. After a year, Adriane missed her family and wanted to move back to California; she was homesick. Joel, Adriane and I moved back to California together. Now that I look back, we should have stayed in Rochester.

We were all afraid of becoming lifers at Kodak, as everyone else was. In the day, Kodak Park had everything anyone ever needed. The park was seven miles wide and twelve miles long. They had restaurants, grocery stores, clothing stores, movie theaters, and bowling alleys. The pay and benefits were great but we were not ready for that, not yet. Back to California we went, and for a time lived with Adriane's mom.

Adriane found work with her brother as a machinist. Joel and I could not find decent jobs, so we started cutting wood and selling it by the cord. We never made much money, but we worked like hell anyway. Our party time continued, except that the drinking age in California was twenty-one, and Adriane could not get into the bars with us. This caused problems, of course, because Joel and I were wild together, very wild. We still went to private parties and swap meets (as we called swapping partners). Joel met a woman, Lynn, in the Santa Cruz Mountains, and they hooked up together. Now, we four started to swap partners, also. I know it was very risky behavior. Most of that was Joel's and my idea and the girls went along with it. This started to get out of hand, and everything changed again.

December, 1976

Joel and Lynn went to live and ski at Lake Tahoe. Lynn did not like Joel and me together because of the wild things we did. Later, Adriane and I broke up. I went to live in Lake Tahoe. I loved to gamble. That is another risky behavior. Many times we would throw down our checks on a blackjack hand; win, lose or draw, it did not matter. Besides, the casino would always let us borrow money if we worked for them. We gambled a lot while living there and lost a lot. I managed to save some money, and went to a class to learn how to count cards.

The class was twelve hundred dollars, but it was also guaranteed to learn how to count. The system is very easy to learn, and it was easy to count cards. The only problem was that counting cards is illegal in Nevada. It was very easy to be caught, because the only way counting works is if you bet big on the hands that are in your favor and small when they are not in your favor. Even an idiot could tell when you always bet five or ten dollars on hands you lose, and fifty to one hundred on the hands that you win. For the most part, they would just ask you to leave the casino. Soon there would be no place left to play black jack. Even when they used six decks of cards, you could still win and come out ahead. The system never changed.

Irresponsible in Carson City

While living in Lake Tahoe, Joel and I would frequent Carson City and the Mustang Ranch or the Kit Kat club. Joel was doing some plumbing repairs for Joe, who at that time owned the Mustang Ranch. That experience was one I will never forget. Joe paid everybody the same way: cash, drugs or women.

We had fun there. When you walked in, all of the women would line up around the room and introduce themselves. You could sit and chat for a while, or select any one of them. They would bring us drinks, and we could just sit and talk to them. That was nice. It made the whole thing more personal.

After you made your selection, they would take you into one of the many bedrooms. Then you could drink, talk and snort a little coke. You could spend as much time as you wanted with them; after all, it was your dime. I think it was thirty dollars an hour, plus whatever you worked out with the girls. It was a good deal, but, a few times, we left with no money at all.

I remember one time we both drank excessively and we had to drive back to Lake Tahoe. The road was very straight and nothing around but high desert, I mean nothing. Somehow, I fell asleep, and Joel pulled over and went to sleep. This was about two or three in the morning. We woke up at about noon. It was in the nineties. Outside, the sun was beating down on the car.

We had the windows rolled up and it must have been one hundred and thirty degrees in the car. We were both sweating, and could hardly wake up at all. Joel managed to open the door and the heat outside felt very cool. We climbed out of the car, and realized we had no water. We were scorched from the heat, we had no water, and Joel remembered he ran out of gas the night before. And, if that wasn't enough, we were broke with only sixty cents in change. We had no gas can, anyway. I was ready to drink the radiator water. The alcohol from the night before had dehydrated us and we were dying for water.

I had the worst hangover I have ever experienced in my life, and we had to hitch hike back to Lake Tahoe to get money. Everyone was going seventy-five miles an hour, and did not want to stop for us. We actually had to stop cars to get a ride back. We learned a good lesson about being responsible. We were crazy together, Joel and I. There seemed to be chemistry between us whenever we got together. It is almost as if a third person emerged from us, a person much different from either one of us. We were much different alone than we were together, I cannot explain what happened. Maybe we were both bipolar.

We competed with each other and did things that we would not do alone. In Lake Tahoe, we would have a few drinks and then get real balls-y, as we called it. We loved to ski fast and race each other. One time, we were off the trail, as we always were, and before we knew it, we flew off the side of the mountain and across Highway 50, and landed into a snow bank on the other side of the highway. A truck going up the hill to Lake Tahoe almost hit us. Joel broke his right arm and I broke three fingers, though it could have been much worse. It took two months before we could ski again. We decided that drinking that much was not a good idea when we were downhill skiing. Adriane came to Lake Tahoe to ski and be with us. We were separated at that time. The party started again. Yes, we partied hearty. Adriane's mom, Betty, was going through her change of life at that time. Her husband drank all the time.

When Betty would drink, she would come onto Joel and me. We both said we would not give in to her, but one night I got drunk with her, and we had sex. We broke up soon after that. That was the end of Adriane, and the end of our marriage. I moved to Oregon and Adriane stayed in California. She soon filed for a divorce. Our marriage was over. There was nothing I could do to fix it. I lived in McMinnville, Oregon, with Charles Jr.; McMinnville is a college town. I met and slept with more women there than anywhere else I lived. The drinking and the parties continued, but only in a different place with different people.

My brain seemed to speed along faster than the other people around me. I bought cars, but failed to pay for them; I would get a job, and be fired or quit. I have had more different jobs than anyone else I have ever met. I could not keep my mouth shut, and when things did not go my way, I had no problem telling people what I thought. I started hundreds of different things but never finished them; my brain would go on to something else.

My credit was destroyed from losing jobs, and not being able to make the payments on what I bought. I got more speeding tickets than anyone else I knew. I would drive 55 miles an hour, and within a minute, I would look at the speedometer and I would be doing 70. I would slow to 55 again and within a very short time, I was doing 70 again. I could not control my speed, and I was pulled over for speeding all the time. I lost my license several times over this. When I had a car with cruise control that worked, it would help a lot, if I remembered to set it.

Charles Jr. decided to go to Houston, Texas for contract work as a painter. He asked me to go, and I did. The gypsy in me always wanted to roam. The small town we were in was in a dry county. That meant there were no bars or liquor stores there. However, you could join a private club for thirty-five dollars a week and drink in someone's home that was converted into a bar. You had to bring your own liquor, and buy the setup from the bar. In other words, they supply the glass, ice and soda for two dollars, and you supplied the alcohol. What a racket they had. You could buy liquor in another county that was only six miles away, though. Every weekend was the same thing. The people there would work their ass off, go out and get drunk, then get into a fight, of course, and spend the night at a motel with any woman who came along.

These people were crazy by my standards. The house we painted was actually two houses equaling ten thousand square feet. The house was built by a preacher who happened to find oil on his land. He had a big oil well pumping oil, twenty-four hours a day, from his back yard. The house was actually two homes: one for his family and one for his parents. When we returned to McMinnville, I stayed a short while, and then left for Alaska.

ALASKA AGAIN
March, 1978

The Trans-Alaska Pipeline had started up, and I wanted to be there. In Fairbanks, the Alaska Pipeline Service Company hired me as a painter through the union. My job was to paint the inside of the pump stations. The minimum workday was twelve hours, but it was more like sixteen hours a day, for three to six months. My starting pay was forty-five dollars an hour. The overtime grossed me over five thousand dollars a week.

The Pipeline had no law or order. It was like the Wild West. We were paid by check which we would then cash on the North Slope. There were people running around with tens of thousands of dollars in cash. Drugs were everywhere, mostly cocaine. We had bars just like any other town and whores everywhere. The poker pots were in the tens of thousands. People were shot, robbed and killed. It was wild. I fit right in there, because there was no law and order. One thing about me is that I am rebellious, and I hate to be told what to do.

After a few murders, the Feds came in and took away all the drugs and alcohol. All that did was raise the price for black market drugs and alcohol. Vodka went from twenty-five dollars a fifth to fifty. Most of the whores were welders. They trained in welding so they could get on the North Slope. Whoring was how they made all their money. I and another person offered one of the girls five hundred dollars for both of us, and she laughed at us and told us to come back when we had some money.

The Feds took away the whores; and the ability to cash our paychecks. The checks had to be sent to some other place rather than the North Slope, like to a family member or a bank somewhere. We were only allowed twenty-five dollars every week for necessities. In addition, we could only stay up there for three weeks, and then we had to be home for three weeks. In other words, they totally screwed up any fun we had.

I will never forget the big banner stretched across Main Street in Fairbanks. It said, "God grant me one more pipeline. I promise not to piss this one away". Many people left the North Slope broke and totally burned out, and I was one. I left the pipeline with a few thousand dollars, a car and a motorcycle. I came back to the lower forty-eight, and stopped by Spokane to see a friend I had made while in Alaska named Dennis. Dennis and I partied a lot on the pipeline, so when we got back together it was fireworks. When I came down from Alaska, I had thousands of dollars. Dennis also had money from the pipeline. When I hooked up with Dennis, we rented a suite in the Camlin Hotel. We partied and had many people who were friends, or at least we thought they were. We stayed at the Camlin for three days and did nothing but party. There were all different kinds of drugs, women and alcohol. I counted fifty people, give or take. We had room service and a tab at the bar downstairs.

Dennis had a good friend at the party who was an attorney. He was the keeper of our cash. On the third day, I woke up, and everyone was gone except Dennis and myself. We found out that our room service charges ran an average of twenty-five to thirty-five dollars an hour, and ran for thirty-six consecutive hours. Our tab at the bar was almost seven hundred dollars. The suite was over five hundred dollars a night.

The sleazy attorney took off with the money and was nowhere to be found. We did not have any choice at this point. We had to leave. The hotel had the MasterCard that belonged to Dennis, which did not even come close to covering what we owed. We grabbed our clothes, and out we went down the street. At that time, Dennis lived with his father and that was where we went. We came up with a way to make money from our experience in Alaska.

There were many people in Spokane who wanted to make good money and wanted to work on the pipeline. The problem was that many people never had the opportunity, mainly because they had no contacts. They would go to Alaska and leave broke without a job. What we did was give them the information they needed to get a job for a price. We ran ads in the newspapers and had many people contact us. We supplied the names of the people who could actually hire them, and charged them between three hundred and five hundred dollars for this information. Our information was factual, and they could be hired before they went to Fairbanks. Of course, they also had to pay the supervisor who hired them. That part we did not get involved in. That was between the supervisor and the employee. It was corruption, of course, but the entire pipeline was corrupt. We did pay back the hotel all the monies we owed them.

The buyers on the pipeline would order giant earthmovers, which cost a few hundred thousand dollars. The earthmovers never made it to the North Slope, and someone made a lot of money. The roads were so bad in areas that if a giant earthmover sank into the road, they just left it there and put the road over it. I heard that, in one place, they lost three earthmovers, stacked one on the other, and they are still there to this day.

Dennis and I partied hearty in Spokane. We were both into shooting drugs, because nothing felt as good as a needle. Besides, it was risky business for bipolar people. We shot mostly coke, but there was a lot of meth, also. The high was incredible. No one would understand the feeling unless they tried it.

The problem is that a year or so later, the euphoria begins to degrade your mind, so that what used to seem wrong was not. That led to many serious problems for anyone shooting drugs. The problem was that I never saw it coming, and neither did Dennis. I caught hepatitis C from Dennis. I did not know what that was, and for twenty-six years, it never bothered me.

There were many medical reasons why the virus hepatitis C did not hurt me, including my DNA makeup, which is a Gnome type 2. My body was able to fend off the damage done by the virus. What the virus does is destroy the liver. Between drinking massive amounts of alcohol and contracting the virus, I should have died from severe liver damage. My liver kept on working, though, and healed itself. I could write a book just on this alone, but that is a whole other thing.

I have a very special relationship with Jesus and God. I truly am believer in the Lord. I do not know how to explain this, but He has always been there for me. Once I accepted Jesus as my Lord and savior, everything changed for me. God has answered my prayers many times and He showed me that He answered them. There was no doubt in my mind at all He answered my prayers. No matter how bad things were for me, He has always been there and everything has worked out for me. I know without any doubt whatsoever that God watches over me and takes care of me.

I dodged the draft. At the time, there was a draft for the Army because of the Vietnam War. When I turned eighteen, the Army found me. Imagine that. I was on my way to Canada, as were all good conscientious objectors who did not want to go to Vietnam and kill people, burn villages and kill woman and children, or be killed. The government gave me choices. One was to go to join the Army and go to Vietnam. The second choice was to go to jail; the third was to work for the government. It did not take long to make that decision.

Off I went to work for the government. They sent me to Alaska. They had plans for me, as well as many others. I wound up scraping I-beams under the barracks on the D.E.W. (distant early warning system) line at forty degrees below zero. We also painted the radar screens, which pointed toward Russia. With silver, rust-inhibitive paint, these radar screens were the equivalent of a football field turned on its edge and curved.

The government was supposed to turn off the radar seventy-two hours before we went out to paint the screens. Instead, they turned the screens off only twenty-four hours before we painted them. We could taste a metallic taste in our mouths when we went out there. Besides that, there were many dead birds at the base of the screen, from flying too close to the screens. I did not realize it at the time, but the radiation had sterilized me. I found this out when Adriane and I tried to have a baby. I was tested and found to have dead sperm. The only way this could have happened was from a large dose of radiation.

DELAROSA COSTANZA

July, 1986

My life really started when I met Delarosa Costanza. Before that, I really did not have any idea what life was really all about. It was 1986. I remember well.

I had returned from Alaska to the Bay Area via Spokane. I looked in the newspaper for a job, and called on an ad that I had seen for a painter. The man's name was Allen. He needed a painter to help with some painting on his home, and a few side jobs that he had. I went to see him, and I was hired.

As I was painting his dining room, a woman came over to visit with him about business; real estate, I think. That was Delarosa. She was pretty, and I was attracted to her, as she was to me. Delarosa had a very professional appearance and speech. I could tell that she had a good education. We drank some wine and talked.

Allen had a hot tub in the backyard, and we all decided to go in. We all kept our clothes on and enjoyed the hot tub. I think we both had a little too much wine. That, along with the hot water, made both of us very high. We started to talk and before long, we were making out and then having sex. I knew that she was not the kind of woman to have sex with someone she had just met. I respected her for that. In the morning, she gave me her phone number and a couple of days, later I called her. She invited me over.

Opposites do attract and we were about as opposite as any two people could be. Where she was very responsible, I was not. When I took risks, she did not. While she was financially sound, I was not. While I enjoyed life, she was busy working and building a future for herself. She worked very hard all of her life. She owned her own home, and owned a rental property besides. She was divorced from a verbally abusive husband and lived alone in San Jose, California. We were attracted to each other, and soon we were living together.

Delarosa had never been on a motorcycle before she met me. I talked her into going for a ride, and reluctantly she climbed on the back of the bike. I could feel how tense she was, and she held on for dear life. It did not take long before she became relaxed and enjoyed riding.

After a few long rides, Delarosa decided to get her own motorcycle. It was a Honda 350, small, and low enough for her to learn on. I think it was the next season when she upgraded to a 650. Delarosa was hooked on riding, and we had a blast together. She liked the people we met while riding, and became part of the biker world. Every weekend we would ride. Delarosa never spent her money on things to enjoy. She had a sensible car and a practical home. I showed Delarosa how to spend money on things to enjoy in life. We went out to dinner, movies, and shopping. It was difficult for me to find a decent job and for the most part, I earned far less than she did.

Her career was paying off as she climbed toward one hundred thousand dollars a year. After going along like this for a year we talked, and decided that I should go to school. I had to get my GED first. Then I went on to community college, and studied computers. I wanted to become a network engineer and design networks.

Delarosa supported me all through school, and when I graduated, it made her so happy. It was not long before I climbed to an annual six figure income. She loved me very much, and I loved her. After my internship, I started to make decent money in Silicon Valley.

Although the stress of living in the bay area kept getting worse, we hung in there. The infrastructure of the bay area had not expanded along with the explosion of Silicon Valley. On average, my commute was two to three hours each way, on the freeways. Sometimes I was so anxious about driving home from work; I would stop and have a few drinks before driving home. Delarosa's commute was far less than that, but the stress of getting to work and home wore on her as well.

My bipolar condition: well, it was alive and well. I think what Delarosa was attracted to was my risky life style. I loved to scuba dive, and I eventually talked Delarosa into going down under. She was terrified, and did not enjoy it at all. I never stopped, when I had the chance. In some parts of Mexico, you can dive without being certified. You can go down to fifty or sixty feet. I loved it. I also liked to skydive. In California, I jumped nine times. It is an incredible feeling. I never considered jumping as risky. Many people have jumped. I also love to parasail. I was never afraid to take chances. I never considered being afraid. I just did these things.

We talked about Delarosa doing these things, but I never got her to try anything except for scuba diving. I would fly and dive within fifteen hours, and people told me that would kill me, but it never did. I was also very spontaneous about doing things. She had to plan everything out.

Delarosa had planned to go to Hong Kong, and I decided to go with her. Hong Kong was a great experience. At that time, Hong Kong was still under British rule. Shortly after that, it went back to China. We took a tour of communist China. That was an eye-opening experience for us.

China was definitely a third world country. The people there lived like animals. The toilets were an open trench, with outhouses placed over the trench. It was gross, to say the least. In China, the people ate what they called thousand-day-old eggs. They would bury eggs in the ground, dig them up, and eat them. The eggs were black, and they seemed to be a sort of drug for these people. They all got high and laughed as they rolled around the floor of the train we were on. We were offered some of the eggs, but we turned them down. Hong Kong itself was great. The shopping was incredible. The people in Hong Kong could duplicate anything you brought to them, especially jewelry.

The only real problem I had with Delarosa was that she's a perfectionist, as was her mother. This made my life with her unbearable, at times. I was far from a perfectionist. In fact, I was just the opposite.

My temper came out a lot while we were living together. It seemed to get worse with time, and I could not control it. I would smash things against the wall if I had a problem with it.

When I was in college, one of my internships was telephone technical support. I worked for a local computer manufacturer, and answered the telephone calls for people who bought the computers and needed technical support. At that time, we also supported the operating system, which was Windows 3.1, one of the first Windows operating systems. Windows had many problems. The software had been released before all the bugs were worked out. When customers called Microsoft at that time, they had to wait between one and three hours before they actually got through to a technician. The computer manufacturers had to provide this service. Otherwise, the end user would return the computer to the store where they bought it. The average wait for a technician was about an hour. I soon realized that many of the calls we received were from businesses that purchased the PC's, and needed help fast when they had a problem.

Our First Business

I talked to Delarosa about starting a new business. I explained to her that a business that was dependent on computers would be willing to pay to get the computer up and running. They could not afford to be down. This was before anyone charged for technical support. I explained that the 900 lines were grossing millions each month for charging three dollars a minute for sex calls. This was a fact as I read the reports on the 900 lines. What I suggested was for us to start a 900 line for technical support. I was way ahead of my time as this was years before anyone thought of charging for support. The way this would work is companies would call a 900 number; we had to answer the phone calls by the third ring as the people who called were being charged three dollars a minute as the phone rang. The difference was that we would have fifty to one hundred techs ready to take calls depending on the call volume.

Delarosa decided to invest in the Startup Company as well as a friend named Allen. I supplied the day to day operations of our call center. Yes, we did receive phone calls and we hired a person to do the marketing of our service. We soon realized that computer manufacturers and the stores that sold the PC's wanted us to take their phone calls. The end user would buy a computer and the technical support was built in for twenty five dollars which the customers never realized. The customer would call an 800 number and that call was directed to our office for a technician. We were paid twenty dollars for every call we took regardless of the outcome. This was outsourcing technical support and we started all that years before anyone else.

The idea and the business plans were perfect for that time. As it turned out we needed money for advertising and for someone to market our idea to the manufactures and stores. Allen agreed that after we started the business he would invest more money to keep the business going. Allen figured hundreds of people would call us without the necessary advertising. He refused to invest more money and Delarosa lost her investment and we lost the business. In the years since then everyone charges for technical support. Microsoft started outsourcing their support calls to a third party that could have been us. Delarosa and Allen argued and fought over his broken promises but the business was gone. Delarosa blamed me for talking her into starting the business; as did Allen. It was a sound business idea and it would have worked.

Things were different between Delarosa and me after that. There was a gap or coldness between us that never really went away. This hurt me deeply;

not so much that she blamed me, but that she lost her money. That pain I felt never went away. I wanted so much to make it up to her but I never could. I lived with that guilt for a very long time as I felt I should for what I did to her. I am a very sensitive person. I cry a lot for a man.

That pain inside of me hurt so much that I started doing drugs again. Cocaine and alcohol seemed to help. I was shooting the Coke and drinking like a fish. Delarosa knew what was going on but she said nothing to me. I would climb into bed and my heart would be beating like a drum at three times the normal speed as I tried to sleep. If I were her I would have said or done something; but she didn't. The stress of living in the Bay Area was getting to us both and we discussed it often. One day I told Delarosa about a place I had been to on my way down from Alaska; Spokane, Washington.

Time went by and I kept talking about Spokane. One day in the summer we planned a motorcycle trip to Spokane. We packed up the bikes and off we went. We stayed in motels at night and drove all day long. It was an adventure as always on a motorcycle we both enjoyed the trip and arrived in Spokane safe and sound. I think we spent a week there and saw all of the city and surrounding areas. Delarosa fell in love with Spokane. Compared to San Jose it was heaven.

Coeur d' Alene, Idaho was only 30 miles away and there was a world class resort area nearby. People complained about the traffic there and Delarosa and I would laugh and say, they don't know what traffic is. We both fell in love with Spokane and decided to move there. It took us seven years to actually make the move. While in San Jose we took many trips on the bikes to Lake Tahoe, Yosemite, Yellowstone, Las Vegas, Santa Cruz and many other places. We enjoyed our lives despite my drugs and alcohol.

I had always cooked throughout my life and did most of the cooking for both of us. I loved to cook and she did not. That was alright with me. Delarosa loved me bipolar and all. Eventually the pain of the failed business went away. I bought a lot of the things that gave us pleasure stereos large TV's fun things like dinners and of course drinks lots of drinks. This started to cause problems between Delarosa and me because I did not give her a check that said for rent or for utilities. She did not count that as helping out, no matter what I bought or paid for things. But I just wanted to have fun and live the good life.

SPOKANE

January 1997

The time came to move to Spokane. I looked on the internet and newspapers for employment in Spokane. Delarosa also checked out the cost of living there and real estate. I found a job, Bank of The America's acquired first national bank and they had a branch in Spokane. There was also the credit card center for Bank of The America's, and a call center for customer service. The call center employed over three hundred people at the time. The bankcard center had very old, outdated computer systems and needed someone to update the network. They flew me to Spokane for an interview. I explained to them that a Microsoft server and operating system for all computers would be a good idea and bring them into the newest technology. They agreed and two weeks later, I was hired.

I moved to Spokane first; it was 1997. Delarosa stayed behind in California and took care of her business there. Delarosa drove up to Spokane so we could look for a house to buy. We spent days looking but could not find the right house. Delarosa was getting ready to go back to San Jose when we received a call from a Real Estate woman whom I had talked to weeks earlier.

She told us about a house that met all of our requirements. We went to look at the house and as soon as we saw it, we knew then that we wanted that house. It was perfect in every way. The house was new and was on the market for two hundred fifty thousand. The house had three thousand square feet finished and an unfinished full basement, which was one thousand square feet for a total of four thousand square feet.

This house would cost over a million dollars in the bay area. We knew it would go up in price; way up. One of the requirements for this house was wall space. We had Bill Mac artwork that was life size so the walls had to accommodate art that was 5 foot five inches long and three feet tall. This was the house. I kept working and Delarosa started the moving process. She packed everything herself which was a bad idea because she had so many collectables to pack. It took her over a month to pack everything. Then she had a moving company pick everything up and move it to Spokane.

My job with Bank of The America's was almost intolerable. The other associates were afraid of change and this made my job almost impossible. The operating system they were using was Novel and an old version of Novel. The outdated system had to go and the new one had to be implemented. No one there knew anything about Microsoft. It was then that I realized I do not play well with others and I do not. My manic side would lash out at people because they refused to learn the new system. They made me the bad person. I was the devil behind all these changes and they did not like me at all. Security was the big issue as customer records had to be protected. Although I didn't care what they thought of me, I felt that I did not have the support of management and I was on my own. This seemed unfair to me because I had no real authority over anyone. I would tell people what had to be done and they did whatever they wanted to while management did nothing to help me. I was told when I was hired that I would work closely with Steve who implemented the Novel in the first place. That never happened and we were working against each other all the time. I did not hold back on what I said to management. The way I looked at the situation was, as they were not doing their job; I could not do mine. It was that simple. The other employees laughed at me because they knew that they did not have to listen to me. This was not a good working relationship for anyone who is bipolar. I came down on everyone who was in my way. When I did go to management for help they did not seem to care, I could not understand why.

Time went on and we moved into our new home. At that time, it was winter and very, very cold. While in San Jose, Delarosa and I had opened our home to thirteen Farrell cats. We would catch the cats, take them to the vet, give them their shots, have them fixed, and release them again. The problem was that we were both animal lovers and fell in love with the cats. As a result we ended up keeping thirteen of them. During the move, Delarosa drove to Spokane in a rented van with all thirteen cats in the back. When she stopped at a motel all the cats went in with her. When she left the motel all the cats went in the van again. She did not want them to get cold in the van.

While Delarosa was packing, I was busy finishing the basement of our new home. I explained to Delarosa that I always wanted a bar in my home. Not just a wet bar but a real bar. Well this basement had the perfect place to build a bar and I had it all figured out in my mind what needed to be done. After Delarosa made it to Spokane the basement became our first major project of many. The only way I could concentrate and get projects finished was to have three or four projects going at once. When I was bored with one project, I would jump to another project. The bipolar person becomes disinterested very easily and usually will not finish projects they have started.

This was one project I did finish. In the end, the actual bar was eighteen feet long with a natural stone top. The walls of the bar were made glass blocks that had lights behind them that lit up the blocks. Behind the bar was another bar, the back bar which was also a natural stone top. Behind the back bar were smoked mirrors and glass shelves that hung from that back wall with all the liquor bottles displayed. Behind the front bar was all the necessary equipment to make it a real bar. Even today, I do not know how I did it. It was perfect in every way and I did it with no plans at all except in my mind. I found bar mirrors, neon lights, beer signs, and even some nostalgic lighted pictures. On the back bar sat all the glasses and stem ware on top of lighted clear plastic boxes.

This bar was the best in Spokane. The room itself was sixty feet by forty feet. We built a wine cellar and covered it with brick so it would hold the right temperature. Above the front bar were illuminated glass racks that held all the nice wine glasses. All the lights had dimmers on them for ambiance. We had seating at the bar for twelve and seating in the bar room for twenty more. There was a big screen TV that I built into the wall and a TV set at the bar. We had a Harmon Kardon surround sound system with twelve speakers. The floor was a hearty laminate flooring to withstand the wear of the traffic around the bar area.

The bathroom in the bar was twelve by fifteen feet. The entire bathroom was done in early roman style. There were pillars, which went from the ceiling to the floor, and behind them was a wall-to-wall mural of ancient roman angels. All the fixtures were early European and all the counter tops were natural stone. There was a giant mirror over the pedestal sink. In addition, in one corner of that room was a built in dishwasher for party cleanup. There was a chair rail around the room made of ceramic tile in early roman style. All the lighting was on dimmers. It was magnificent to see. As I said, I do not know how we did that, but we did. It was during that time when I lost my job. Bank of the America's was bought out by National bank and they laid off two hundred and fifty people; I was one of them. Now I understood why everyone had acted as they did. They knew about the merger and never told me. National bank tried to deny my unemployment insurance. When the department of labor found out they flat out told them no! You will pay his unemployment claim.

I wanted to sue the bank for hiring me and moving us to Spokane then laying me off. As they knew about the merger, they did not hire me in good faith. They settled for an undisclosed amount of money. Since I was unemployed, I spent all my time working on the basement. This was eight to twelve hours every day. I built a display case for Delarosa's dolls. It was made of solid oak with mirrors covering the entire back wall and sliding glass doors with glass shelves. In addition, the showcase had many lights that illuminated all the dolls. The display case was twenty-five feet long and from the floor to the ceiling. The display case was a work of art and I don't' know how I pulled that off either.

I was happy doing that kind of work I loved it. I did not know that it would someday bite me in the ass. I did all of the electrical plumbing and building of the entire basement. With so many bar lights, we had to put in heavier wire and higher rated breakers on dedicated circuits. Not to mention all the wiring for the surround system large screen TV and stereo amps to power twelve speakers. I had purchased a Harmon Kardon 5.1 surround sound system for around four thousand dollars. This system had five discreet amplifiers and rated 100 watts per channel. However, this was not RMS watts it was pure power, which is much different. As an example, the volume starts out at minus 70db and goes to 70db plus, a range of 140db. I could never even get the system to minus 0 and start going up to 70plus. At this point, the entire house would shake just like an earthquake. The neighbors would be able to hear the music a full block away. This system was THX certified that means it met or exceeded the sound systems in movie theaters.

In addition to the electrical wiring, we added telephone lines, Dish Network cables, and outdoor lighting for all the gardens as well as outdoor speakers. We put in a suspended ceiling, which I had never done before. The suspended ceiling was to be no more than three inches from the ceiling itself. That was almost an impossible task, especially when you have never done that before. I felt a lot of stress while working on the basement. Remember that I said Delarosa was a perfectionist? If something were off even a sixteenth of an inch, she would complain and have me fix it. I was dealing with a basement where nothing was square within that tolerance. In fact, the basement is where they really do not care if the walls are square or not. I had to deal with that every day. We had many parties in that basement and entertained tens of dozens of people there. We were known for our parties and our bar. Our neighbors were in awe of what we had done in the basement.

Delarosa became critical of everything because I was far from perfect. I started to drink more and more as I could not deal with the stress. I remember when we completed the bar we sat at the bar and had drinks and I still was in awe of what we had accomplished. I could not believe it myself. I was unaware that Delarosa was always worried about my earning money because she never told me that. I just kept working on the house one project after another after another. We fought and argued a lot and I would lash out at her and say many things that I really did not mean. I was vicious and tore into her with all my manic power. I did not want to hurt her, but at the same time I could not handle the pressure I was under. It seemed I could not do anything right no matter how hard I tried. I did look for work during this time but I was always over qualified for the jobs in Spokane. The Bank of The America's paid me fifty two thousand a year, which was a lot of money for the Spokane area. The only jobs that were available in the computer field paid between ten and thirteen dollars an hour and they would not hire me because they could not come close to paying me the wage that I used to make. I became frustrated and stopped applying for jobs in the computer field. I started to look for sales jobs because I knew I could sell.

Doing all the work on the house was difficult for me because my mind would wonder and I could not focus on any one thing very long. I had to concentrate on what I was doing because I had many different projects going at the same time. I lost my temper hundreds of times while working on the house. I tried not to destroy things but sometimes I could not control that. One of our projects was to tear off the rear deck and redo the deck using Trex. I never did that before either but I learned what to do, I also asked many questions. It was mid-summer then, I was working in direct sunlight, and the temperature was in the ninety-degree range. All the work was a labor of love and it took everything I had to complete the projects before me. I would have appreciated a pat on the head or Delarosa telling me what a good boy I was, but she was unable to stop being so critical of me. That bothered me tremendously. All I wanted was a compliment or a "That a boy!" occasionally. The work I did on that house was nothing less than a miracle. I was so busy and there was so much to do that I could not look for work anyway.

Delarosa was always a gardener and she loved it. The entire back yard we turned into gardens. We had mounds filled with perennials on one side and a built up wall all across the back of the yard filled again with perennials. It was a gardener's paradise. I think I counted over three hundred perennials. This did not include the front yard. There was no lawn in the back of the house just gardens. The sprinkler system itself cost hundreds of dollars and was a monumental task. I had to place sprinklers under city sidewalks. I counted over one thousand feet of sprinkler lines. Then of course, the garden had to be cared for and although this was fun, it was a tremendous amount of work for both of us. We tried to build our own waterfall in the back yard.

We rented a backhoe and away we went. When we were done, we were not happy with the waterfall so Delarosa paid thirty two thousand dollars to have one built. This also included the pavers for a patio in the back and a walkway in the front. The waterfall was a thing of beauty. Several thousand gallons of water poured over the falls every few minutes. You could hear the water flow from the street hundreds of feet away. The falls looked so natural that people would swear it was there when they built the house. There were two different falls into one big pond. The pond held over a thousand gallons of water and was four feet deep. The falls had to have a drain hole that was five feet deep and five feet across. This drain was filled with small rocks then ground cover to hide the hole. Periodically the waterfall had to be emptied and refilled again. The total amount of water was over five thousand gallons. Trees lined the falls so all you could see was the falls in a forest of trees. It was incredible. We were on many garden tours where hundreds of people would pay to see our gardens.

The Neighbors

February, 1998

Working on the house and trying to live the life of illusion put a lot of pressure on me and my bipolar was becoming worse with time. I actually started to talk to myself. This may have been an escape from the stress of trying to be perfect. I do not know. I repeated myself over and over again. I could not control that either. I know that Delarosa spent many thousands of dollars on the house but that is what she wanted. Delarosa always made me aware of the money she was spending. I did not know what to say to her. I was doing all that I could do and I never charged her anything for the work I had done and that was many thousands of hours. I was not doing drugs but I did drink a lot. I was looking for some way to feel better about what I was doing. Some of our neighbors became jealous of what we had. Even still, everyone in the neighborhood came to our parties. We were the who's who of South Hill, the rich area of Spokane. Now that I look back at what we were doing, it was very much keeping up with the Jones's and passing them by.

One of our neighbors had extremely bright outdoor lights. Their house was higher than ours was because it was built on a hill. At night, we would sit in the living room and look out at the beautiful waterfall that was lit up with lights that brought the waterfall to life in the dark. The lights on the waterfall were set so no one could see them except us. Our neighbor would turn on their lights, which must have been five hundred watts each and destroyed our ability to see our backyard. Then he would stand on his deck and just look at us. Being the bipolar person that I was I went to the garage and pulled out two construction lights that were one thousand watts each and shined the lights on their house. This was war and I was not going to let them win. This went on for a couple of weeks and escalated. I would stand on our deck and look back at him but nothing changed.

Finally, I went over to the neighbor's house to talk with them and see if we could end this competition that had been going on between us. I knew that the woman who lived there was younger than the man, but I did not know how much until she answered the door. She had to be twenty years younger than he was. She came to the door and was surprised to see me there. She asked me to come in and I did. We sat at the kitchen table as I spoke about the tension. As we talked, I realized that she was a good-looking

47

woman and I wondered why she was with this old man. When I looked around, I knew why; the old man had money. As we talked, she made it clear that she disagreed with the way her husband was reacting. We finished our conversation with an agreement that she would try to get her husband to stop with the lights and I agreed to put away the construction lights. When I left, she smiled at me and thanked me for coming over to talk with her. I figured that was the end of the lights.

Three days went by with no giant searchlights shining on us at night. Then came the day it started again. The old man was standing there on his deck with even more and brighter lights than before. This really pissed me off and I went ballistic. I stood where he could see me and gave him the finger. He just walked away. This escalated again and the war was on. This time I just stood there and stared at him. His wife was not involved as far as I could see. The next night I was drinking and he turned on his lights. I was so pissed off that I pulled down my pants and showed him my ass. Delarosa was out of town at that time. He walked away again. I thought that might stop him. I noticed his wife was watching me. I pulled up my pants and left the room but she remained there watching. This went on for days and I realized she was interested in what I was doing. I found a player and she definitely was interested. Delarosa traveled a lot for her job and she was away from home a lot. This woman had to be desperate for something exciting in her life and it was not her husband. When I went to her house, she had told me that he was a doctor.

As a doctor, he was gone a lot evenings and like me, she was home alone. One time her husband came home and noticed that she was watching our house, I had left the window instantly when I saw him. I did not think that he had seen me and I left it at that. We both stopped for a while. Then came the day when she was standing at the window watching our house. I was looking at her and she smiled at me, the game was on. I know a lot of you who are reading this book may be asking yourselves, "Why did I continue doing this. Why did I not stop this game or why didn't she stop it?" The answer is the same for both of us; there were great rewards both mentally and physically. If there were not some kind of reward, we would not have played the game. I did not need any drugs, just alcohol and I noticed she always had a glass of wine throughout the entire evening. This went on for two years. I knew that if she really did not want to see me she could close the drapes. She never did that. I would like to mention that one should repeat what I did. Even if two people are exhibitionist in nature, there may be serious legal penalties for doing this, as I will explain.

A woman can play this game for years and one day call the police and tell them that you are watching her. It is the same as a woman having sex with you and then one day calls the police and tells them that you raped her. No matter what the circumstance; she is right and you are wrong, exhibitionism is illegal. Would it not seem insane to keep doing this knowing the risk involved? Not when you are bipolar and you do very risky things. Can I then justify what I was doing? No, remember earlier I wrote about that the bipolar condition has no logic. This type of action is just what I was talking about. People could say that I could have stopped at any time, that I must be a very perverted person, or that I knew what I was doing and knew that it was wrong. All this may be true but the fact remains that I never weighed the right or wrong and never thought about the consequences while I was doing this.

Then one would have to ask why did the woman not stop this? She could be as sick as I was then or she could be bipolar or even crazy. No matter the reason, the game went on for both of us and she was one of few women who did this. I experienced couples who would watch me as they had sex with each other; I think a lot of this had to do with the fact that this was taboo in our society and there was always a chance of being caught. I am sure that as you read this you would think about people who have sex in an elevator or some other public places where they might be caught. This adds to the thrill of having sex.

Why sex? I cannot answer that question. Sex can be healing and as I said, it takes two consenting adults. Why drugs? Why gambling? Why alcohol? Why a sex addiction? Why to all the crazy things we do in life? If someone did not want to participate in the game, all they had to do is shut the other person out by closing the blinds. It's that simple. If one of us did not feel like playing the game, or had company, we could just close the blinds. Then the legal aspect comes into play. If you did not want to see what was going on then close the blinds. As far as the law is concerned, the question would be why are you watching this? They cannot say that someone was breaking the law if you continue to watch what they are doing. You cannot enjoy the show and then get your money back. It does not work that way.

One day her husband caught her watching me and that was the end of the show. He called the police and told them what was going on. The first thing they asked was how long this had been going on. The reason for that question was simple, that they had this complaint before from the same people two years ago. You cannot cry wolf for two years and then blame the wolf. If her husband had not been a prominent doctor then that was as far as that would go. However, he told her either she presses charges or he would leave and take the children. She had no choice. She did what he wanted or she would lose her family. It was a no brainer. The way the law reads, a woman can watch a man naked man for years and then one day she can decide that she does not want to see him anymore. Then this goes to court with a charge of indecent exposure for the man. (Me). That is what happened. When I went to court, I had a female Judge. I informed the court that I would represent myself. I entered a plea of not guilty. The judge warned me to make sure that

I understood the ramifications of what I was doing. This is because if I was found guilty I could not win on appeal because of having poor representation. I could see that the judge did not want this case in court at all. She acted as if it was a total waste of time. She made that clear to the prosecuting attorney. She had a real bad attitude toward the attorney. She accepted my not guilty plea and set a pre- trial hearing in sixty days.

I had a friend Greg who was a private detective and worked as bounty hunter. I had worked with him on occasion. It was a boring job sitting in a car all night waiting for the person to show so you could cuff them and bring them back to jail. It was mostly women who jumped bail and had Failure-to-Appear warrants out for them however, it did pay well. I had Greg do some discovery work for me. The neighbor's house was three hundred feet away from our house. Their house was higher than ours was. No one in our neighborhood liked this woman at all. All she could talk about was her husband the doctor. Greg learned that they had moved to Spokane from Texas. He also learned that they were separated in Texas because she had an affair. This would hurt her credibility which was good for me. Greg also found out that the prosecuting attorney had been sexually molested as a child and she tried to bury anyone who had any sexual charge.

I filed several motions against the State for evidence they had collected. This kept the case from going to trial for a year. I was representing myself so the DA had to show me the evidence they had against me. Most was circumstantial or hear- say. During this time, I had been diagnosed bipolar. I told my psychiatrist everything that I did and was involved in. She told me she had heard it all before; therefore, when I told her about the game I played she was not surprised at all. I told her about the pending court case and she said that she would provide a copy of my mental condition and explain that I am bipolar. She also told me if that did not work then she would testify on my behalf and I would not have to subpoena her.

On the next court date there was a different attorney for the state. The first motion from the state was to ask for more time to go over the case. The judge denied the request and stated that the State had had sufficient time to prepare. The attorney did not know what to do. I then turned my medical report over to the court and the attorney. The first thing he did was say he objected to my evidence as hear-say. The judge agreed with him. My next motion was for my Psychiatrist to testify for me. The attorney looked surprised and the Judge said OK we have our first expert witness. She looked directly at the attorney. The Judge called us up to the bench for a side bar. She asked the state if they were ready for trial. She used a tone that was more "Do you really want to go ahead with this?" At that point, the attorney said that he would try to offer me a deal on a lesser charge. She agreed and set another trial date. I asked the attorney what he had in mind. He offered indecent exposure, thirty days in jail, and one-year probation with a three hundred dollar fine. I told him no and walked away. The DA was catching dissension from the doctor on why this has not been settled yet.

A few days later the District Attorney called me in and wanted to make another offer. The state knew about my evidence, as I had to turn all my evidence over to them as they did me. Greg found one of our neighbors who would testify that the game went on for two years. I went to the DA's office, sat down with the attorney, and asked him what he was offering. By now, he knew about our neighbor who was willing to testify. He offered indecent exposure, two weeks in jail, no fine and one-year probation. I countered with time served as I was in jail one day already when I was booked in and released; time served, as well as one-year probation and no fine. He said the state will not go for that. I said why not ask them He left the room and when he returned he stated we would have an agreement if I served one more day in jail. I agreed and that was over. We went before the Judge and gave her our decision. She looked it over and with a sigh of relief asked "Do we all agree?" We did and that was that. The one day in jail is actually eight hours. I am sure the good doctor was pissed off about that.

OUR BUSINESS

August, 2004

This was where we made our money in Real Estate and became rich; well for a minute anyway. It was time for me to find a job, any job. I did not care; I needed my own money. I looked in the papers and on the internet. It seemed there was nothing. The jobs I did apply for had thirty other people applying for the same jobs. I was looking in the business section of the newspaper. I saw an ad that offered a soda franchise. That sounded interesting to me so I called the number in the ad. It was True Soda looking for someone to sell and distribute soda beverages in the greater Spokane area. We talked for about an hour. The owner Danny told me where I could find his products in a nearby store. I said that I would check out the beverages and get back to him.

I went to the store. The business was a specialty store that sold mostly organic foods and produce along with hard to find food items. I asked about the specialty soda and everyone acted weird, as I had done something wrong. They were hesitant to show me where the beverages were in the store. As I was checking out the beverages, the beverage manager came over and asked if he could help me. I replied no I was just looking at the beverages, the manager kept watching me as I read the labels. I thought that was somewhat weird, but I kept reading. I noticed the beverages were all in glass bottles and made with pure cane sugar. The packaging was very unique and replicated the classier era of the fifties. I bought a couple of bottles and tasted the soda beverages. The taste was incredible! It was what I remembered from my childhood. I knew that I could sell this soda very easily to supermarkets, c-stores and restaurants. I knew that Spokane was a very conservative place and I would only be able to sell high quality beverages in Spokane.

I took some of these sodas home and showed them to Delarosa she was impressed by the quality and the packaging of these beverages. I explained to Delarosa about the franchise and told her how easy it would be for me to sell these beverages. I bought more of these sodas to show to the managers of The markets. Their reactions to the beverages were very good. They told me that they would carry the beverages in their stores and make twenty five to thirty points on them. When I returned to buy more beverages from the store this young man and woman came over to me and started asking me many questions.

I simply told them the truth about the ad and that I was considering selling the beverages. These people told me all about how bad the owner of the soda franchise was and all the terrible things that he had done to them. They told me how he cost them tens of thousands of dollars. They said he shipped beverages to them that they never ordered and could not sell. I did not know any better and took their word for what they were telling me. I thought about that and told them that I could sell these beverages for them instead of buying a franchise. They thought about this offer and we had a meeting together two days later and agreed that I would sell for them.

When I arrived at their warehouse, we went in and they showed me their products. As I looked around, I could see products that I knew I would never sell. They had beverages with the names Brainwash, Belly Wash, Fukola, Rat Bastard, Leninade and Black Lemonade. I could tell just by looking at the beverages that I could never sell any of them. Spokane was excessively conservative for a product label like these. I knew I could sell a few but I could never sell enough to make a living at it. The only beverage they carried that I knew I could sell was the Boylan brand. So that is what I started selling. I went to all the major markets in Spokane and within thirty minutes, they all ordered from me. Everything was going great when it came time to deliver the beverages to the stores they ran out of Boylan brand. I asked when they could get more and they replied they could not get more. When I asked why they said that they owed Danny fifty thousand dollars and until that was paid, they could not get the Boylan brand.

I talked the stores into stocking Americana soda products instead of Boylan. They agreed and we brought in the Americana sodas. We gave samples out and gave customers a lower price but the soda did not sell. Once people tried the Americana, they would never buy anymore. I could not blame the customers; it tasted like crap. I asked the store I worked for why they owed Danny fifty thousand dollars and the management did not have a clear answer.

I got in contact with Danny, the owner of True Soda, and had a long conversation with him. I found out that everything the management of the market told me was a lie and they did owe Danny the money. They ordered all kinds of soda that they could not sell. They did not know their market at all. When the product failed to sell, management ordered more of the same as before. The beverages sold so slowly that by the time they sold a load, they were out of money.

They begged Danny into shipping them more soda and at the end of the day, they owed fifty thousand dollars and still could not sell their beverages. These people definitely were not business people. I kept Delarosa informed about all that happened and I told her I could place these products in all the major stores. We talked about all the pros and cons of starting the business. We had a sound business plan and I already had customers ready for the beverages. We paid the five thousand dollars for the franchise fee and ordered our first Truckload of beverages.

It was very easy for me to sell the sodas to anyone I talked to. All the markets cared about was how much it would cost and how much they could make. That is all. Delarosa went with me as I sold to all the major markets in the Tri Cities area of Washington. I would walk in the store and I would walk out in less than ten minutes with an order. I did this seven times in one day and they were big orders; at least one pallet for each store which was seventy two cases each. Being bipolar helped me to sell anything to anybody. I was good at selling. I overcame objections in less than thirty seconds flat. Delarosa was as proud of me as I was of myself. The previous owners blamed everyone for their failing business. Everyone that is, except themselves. They filed a lawsuit against us for the name and logo associated with True Soda. That was pointless because the name and logo was not ours; it belonged to Danny in L.A. We retaliated by filing a lawsuit against them. The business insurance covered all of our legal expenses.

The only people who came out ahead on the lawsuit were the attorneys. We did win the rights to use the name and logo of True Soda and they lost the rights. I have learned that you have to keep your friends close and your enemies closer. Our businesses were at war. Every market that we approached about carrying our product, the bastards from the other market would go in and tell management how we screwed them over and stole their soda. They accused us of selling that soda to the stores. They blamed us for everything that went wrong with their business. They also blamed us for them losing fifty thousand dollars. Unfortunately, the managers believed them.

These people were well practiced in the art of deception. Our new marketplace stores did not want to get in the middle of our businesses, so they threw our product out of their stores. Even if the product was thrown away, our enemies considered it a win. They were very destructive and didn't care if that meant we were losing everything. They did not care as long as they destroyed our business. They were going to lose their business and wanted to take us down with them. This caused serious problems with our customers as no one wanted to get in the middle of this battle.

Some of our customers had their own attorneys involved because they did not know what to do about the situation. They could not take us out of the stores for fear of us suing them. However, the other company was also believable. The bastards continued to work on getting us out of all of our stores. Unfortunately, they were very good at what they did. People with bipolar disorder can get very mean, very fast. We are a vicious lot of people. Vengeance is a dish best served cold is our motto and it is true. One time in New York, we had a bully who used to take our money. This happened to me a few times. One day I took my father's knife with me to school. When he came up to me, all I could see was a yellow flash in my eyes. I took the knife and cut up his face bad. The other kids told me that he went to the hospital. A couple of weeks later he came back to school. His face was all scared up.

I did not realize what I had done to him; it was as if I went into a blackout. No one ever told anyone what I did. I found out later that everyone was afraid of me. I had a lot of respect after that. I have been that way all my life. When I had to fight, I would never just punch anyone. I always went for the eyes or the throat. I did not actually know what I did until it was over. I once put my thumbs in some person's eyes and pressed so hard it brought him to his knees and that was the end of the fight even though he was bigger than I was. When I watched television, I always wondered why people would punch each other. It did not make any sense at all, it was stupid. If I could not reach the eyes or the throat, I would grab their testicles and squeeze real hard while as I pulled as hard as I could. I did not think about this. It just happened. As I look back, I can see that my cousin Star was the same way. No one would ever mess with her, including me. We used to joke about getting into a fight and we both agreed that it would be a blood bath and that never happened.

By this time the stress had already overcome me and I felt I was going crazy. My bipolar disorder started to take over my life. I could not control the bipolar and I could not control the business. I felt like everything was coming down around me. Delarosa and I had not had sex for a long time. She was gone most of the time because she traveled frequently for work. This actually made things a lot harder for me because I was alone and had to make many of the decisions myself. In our society, we live for instant gratification even if it lasts only a little while. We have all bought something new like a car and we take better of that car than we take care of ourselves. Soon that new feeling leaves and it is just a car.

The gratification is a fleeting moment in time. For someone who is bipolar that feeling of gratification needs to be repeated time after time. We cannot control that. This could be anything at all. It does not matter what the vice is. Remember this is a case of undiagnosed bipolar, after treatment all of this fades away. What gratification is for us is a means to an end. At the end of the day we never mean to hurt anyone, what we do is not premeditated. Our actions are very spontaneous. However, God help the people who get involved with us. We tear them apart and hurt them beyond imagination. We are very toxic and we can poison any one at any time and not realize what we devastation that I have caused. The only way I can do this is to interview someone who I lived with or was married too. This will not be easy for either of us. However, it is the only way for me to explain what the other person feels and the hell they have lived. You, the reader need to know what it is like living with a bipolar person.

The way I was diagnosed was accidental. I was at the dentist office and I picked up the magazine and started reading it. In the magazine, there was a small survey of twenty questions. I filled out the survey as best I could then I added up the score as instructed. At the bottom of the survey was a sentence that read; if you answered yes to any of these questions you may be bipolar. I looked at the survey and I answered yes to all the questions. It also said that if you did say yes to any of these questions you should bring this survey to your family Doctor. On my next appointment with my Doctor, I brought the survey and showed it to him. The Doctor looked at the survey and said to me that I looked like the poster child for bipolar. The Doctor referred me to a psychiatrist.

When I met with the psychiatrist, she had me take a 600 question test. I took the test and answered all the questions as best as I could. The test took two hours and had to be graded by a third party. It took one month to get the results back. My psychiatrist called me and made another appointment to come in. We sat down and she looked over the scores and she actually said the same thing my family Doctor had said. I was a poster child for bipolar disorder. The tests showed that I was bipolar one. Since then I have been diagnosed three separate times.

That is when I started medical treatment and many counseling sessions. The different medications that we started with had many side effects. During this time, many weird things happened to me. I saw situations and conversations that did not happen. These mimicked symptoms of the mental illness called schizophrenia. At first I thought people were just joking with me, but after talking to a number of different people whom I didn't know, I came to the conclusion that I was seeing things that weren't there and that never happened. There was one other side effect to the medication and that was that I kept repeating myself. I could not control this and it bothered me. When I spoke to my psychiatrist about that, she told me that the medications were battling within my brain as the drugs started to work. It is a period of confusion. During this time I should signs of other mental illness. I could have been diagnosed as schizophrenic or having a personality disorder, or any other number of things. This period of confusion did not last very long. Thank God for that. At this time, I was fifty-eight years old and just diagnosed. As I mentioned earlier in the book bipolar gets worse with time. By the time I was diagnosed bipolar, it had had fifty-eight years to grow. All of this goes along with what I mentioned earlier. are or have been doing to them. In this book, I will try to explain the pain and devastation that I have caused. The only way I can do this is to interview someone who I lived with or was married too. This will not be easy for either of us. However, it is the only way for me to explain what the other person feels and the hell they have lived. You, the reader need to know what it is like living with a bipolar person.

The way I was diagnosed was accidental. I was at the dentist office and I picked up the magazine and started reading it. In the magazine, there was a small survey of twenty questions. I filled out the survey as best I could then I added up the score as instructed. At the bottom of the survey was a sentence that read; if you answered yes to any of these questions you may be bipolar. I looked at the survey and I answered yes to all the questions. It also said that if you did say yes to any of these questions you should bring this survey to your family Doctor. On my next appointment with my Doctor, I brought the survey and showed it to him. The Doctor looked at the survey and said to me that I looked like the poster child for bipolar. The Doctor referred me to a psychiatrist.

When I met with the psychiatrist, she had me take a 600 question test. I took the test and answered all the questions as best as I could. The test took two hours and had to be graded by a third party. It took one month to get the results back. My psychiatrist called me and made another appointment to come in. We sat down and she looked over the scores and she actually said the same thing my family Doctor had said. I was a poster child for bipolar disorder. The tests showed that I was bipolar one. Since then I have been diagnosed three separate times.

That is when I started medical treatment and many counseling sessions. The different medications that we started with had many side effects. During this time, many weird things happened to me. I saw situations and conversations that did not happen. These mimicked symptoms of the mental illness called schizophrenia. At first I thought people were just joking with me, but after talking to a number of different people whom I didn't know, I came to the conclusion that I was seeing things that weren't there and that never happened. There was one other side effect to the medication and that was that I kept repeating myself. I could not control this and it bothered me. When I spoke to my psychiatrist about that, she told me that the medications were battling within my brain as the drugs started to work. It is a period of confusion. During this time I should signs of other mental illness. I could have been diagnosed as schizophrenic or having a personality disorder, or any other number of things. This period of confusion did not last very long. Thank God for that. At this time, I was fifty-eight years old and just diagnosed. As I mentioned earlier in the book bipolar gets worse with time. By the time I was diagnosed bipolar, it had had fifty-eight years to grow. All of this goes along with what I mentioned earlier. I could see the business failing but there was nothing I could do to stop it. It was beyond my control but it still weighed very heavy on my mind. The retail store The Soda Shoppe, averaged one thousand dollars a day profit the first year it was open. Everyone in Spokane wanted to come into our store simply because The Soda Shoppe came back after twenty-one years. It was a type of nostalgia that

Spokane supported. The Soda Shoppe was something that everyone remembered from their childhood. The economy hurt the store and at that point, we had seven employees delivering soda to the markets and running the retail store. I was working sixteen hours a day, seven days a week and could not keep up with the workload. Delarosa was buried doing payroll and working her regular job.

I started to drink a lot and managed to acquire three DUI's, and two hit and runs. One hit and run was while the vehicle was occupied and the next on a non-occupied hit and run. The occupied hit and run went like this; I was going through a green light when out of nowhere came a vehicle that flew through the red light at about fifty miles an hour, the speed limit was thirty. I was doing thirty-five. I hit them and it was like hitting a block wall. I had a Jeep Cherokee that someone had removed the air bags from. I was thrown into the steering wheel and knocked out and I had my seatbelts buckled. When I came to, I was lying on the ground. My car was destroyed.

I tried to walk but I kept falling down. I was in a fog and really did not know how bad the accident was at the time. I wandered off and lay down on some grass about thirty feet from the car. I watched the police and fire rescue trucks arrive. Everyone told the police where I was. The officers did not want to walk over to where I was so they classified the accident as a hit and run. Off to jail I went and of course I had been drinking. The other vehicle was a SUV. They were drunk and had no license and no insurance. They had to be cut out of the SUV with the Jaws of Life. The witnesses told the police what happened but everyone went to jail anyway; imagine that. Both vehicles were totaled. I was in jail for another week. Thank God, no one was hurt.

The other hit and run was a sign a non-occupied sign. I was drunk and it was my fault because I drove off. They caught up with me and off to jail I went another time. I should mention here that I had stopped taking my meds. I was having so many problems with the business and with Delarosa; I just could not cope with the stress. When I stopped taking the meds, I went manic and of course, that made everything worse, but I did feel better.

I hired a woman to work for me at The Soda Shoppe named Stacey who was 25 years old. She was a very beautiful woman who was five foot five with brown hair and blue eyes. She was hired to work in the retail outlet as she brought in many people, mostly men. I did get involved with Stacy and this is something I should not have done. Nevertheless, I could not help myself because she was so beautiful and helped relieve my stress. The only problem with Stacy was that she was a party animal and caused many problems. I really did not need any more problems. I had enough as it was. However, I could not help myself. I felt sorry for Stacey and tried to help her.

By the time I figured out that she was buried in drugs and partying, and that there was no way to help her, it was too late for me. I would let her borrow my truck and she would stay out all night with it. I had to track her down to get my truck back and sometimes that did not work. Stacy was sexually molested as a child by her father. This really screwed her up. Since she already had a personality disorder, this criminal act was devastating to her. She drank more than I ever did and did more drugs than anyone else I knew. Stacy was hooked on prescription pain meds.

When she scored the meds then she would begin to party. These were no ordinary parties. They were incredibly wild even for me. I watched her snort enough cocaine to kill someone. Then her clothes would come off. It did not matter who was there or what sex they were. She would have sex with five to ten people, one after the other. Because her father had molested and raped her, the only way she enjoyed sex is if it hurt her. Stacy had a son (Dominick) who at the time was five years old. Stacey's mother raised Dominick because she could not.

Her mom did not trust her with Dominick and I understood why. Stacy learned at a very young age how to use people to get what she wanted. A prostitute at eighteen, she always used everyone she met; including me. It made me feels good to go places and do things with her because everyone always looked at her wishing they were me. I think that part of this was my second childhood.

One night after work, she asked me if I would buy her a drink and I said, "Yes." She played her cards very well and this was her drug card. After a few drinks, she asked me if I wanted to get high. I asked her, "High on what?" She replied, "Coke, of course." I asked her where we were going to get coke. Stacy informed me that she had some friends we could score from. I agreed and off we went to Post Falls, Idaho. When we arrived, she made a phone call. We had to wait for about twenty minutes. I began to realize what I was getting into and I wanted to say no but I could not, big mistake. When her connection arrived, they parked directly behind us. At this point Stacy said they do not have any coke but they do have meth. I knew I was screwed now and could not turn back. I gave her the money and she scored the meth. Stacy showed me a place where we could park and smoke the meth. I took a couple hits and told her I wanted to go home. She did not want to leave yet. I told her at that point that I was leaving and I could drop her off somewhere. She was like a fiend and just kept puffing on the pipe. She also had a friend in the car from the other vehicle. I dropped her off and she asked if she could keep my share of the meth. I told her yes as I did not need any more of that shit. I dropped her and her friend off and headed home. Anyway, that was Stacy and the party never stopped. She partied more than I ever did. This was a new generation of party animals.

There is a difference between being bipolar, having a personality disorder, or being Schizophrenic. It is a very small, slight difference. The imbalance in the brain is very slight but it makes an incredible amount of difference. As for the sociopath person, we believe that they are monsters. They feel that what they do is normal. To them it is but a game. They do not feel any remorse or guilt for what they do. They do not feel that what they do is bad and the game is not to be caught. It is a game of cat and mouse. The IQ of the average serial killer is very high, in the one hundred seventy to two hundred range. They are very intelligent people.

Ted Bundy was an example. He escaped from maximum-security prison three times. Ted saw things that no one else could see, even the prison guards who had worked there for years. Ted Bundy saw the flaws and weaknesses in the prison system and he took advantage of them. Our society cannot accept the behavior of the sociopath so we put them down. This is a normal reaction for the unimaginable horror that they cause society. We give them a deal of life in prison without parole rather than the death penalty in exchange for the information they have about their victims. Where are the bodies of the victims? One would wonder why the FBI or any branch of law enforcement could not find these bodies.

The answer is that Law enforcement does not have the intelligence of the serial killer and cannot figure out what they might do next. The FBI uses profilers to figure out who serial killers are. They can tell us what their age is and whether or not they are married. They can tell us how many children they have and communities they live. They can tell us what color they are and what nationality they are. They can even tell us what they would have as a hobby. One thing these profilers cannot tell us is why they do this horrible crime. This is beyond the FBI and any profilers. The scientific community has found a gene in the DNA that only sociopathic people have. They have isolated this gene and found this gene in every sociopathic killer. Science has many years of research ahead of them to figure out how to remove this gene from DNA and they may never be able to accomplish that.

The push for lethal injection was promoted by the scientific community so that they have an undamaged brain to study unlike the electric chair or the gas chamber, which causes severe damage to the brain. In addition, lethal injection is more humane. There are traits in the sociopath that always predates any sociopathic activities. Some of these are hurting small animals and children. They seem to get pleasure out of this behavior at a very young age. They can sexually abuse and rape family members. One thing to keep in mind is that there are women who are serial killers. They also have the same traits as the men do and follow the same patterns. We have all heard of the Black Widow who married men and then killed them for their money. Aileen Wuornos is one of many women who were serial killer's and there is a movie made about her case.

The profilers gain much of their knowledge from interviews with the sociopathic killers. Hundreds of hours of painstaking interviews that no one ever wanted to hear or think about. These interviews, no matter how horrifying they were gave great insight into the sociopath. These interviews were a means to an end. Some of the FBI agents had to undergo psychiatric treatment after the interviews that they had conducted. As I said earlier, there is a small difference between these mental conditions and that makes an incredible difference. You may be asking where I am going with all this and what does this have to do with being bipolar. The reason for this is to understand the human brain. Perhaps then we can understand the horror and mayhem that we cause others. This will become apparent to you when I interview someone who has lived with a person who has the bipolar condition.

A person who has lived with someone who is bipolar will never understand bipolar and they will never believe that the bipolar person did not intentionally try to hurt them or destroy their lives. They cannot accept the carnage that we create as being a mental illness. Conversations that I have had with Adriane and Delarosa will prove this point. They have a tremendous hatred toward the person who has caused all this pain in their lives, which is understandable. I could no more control what I did than I could control the weather. No matter how insane this might seem, it is true. The victim will never understand this fact and they will always blame the bipolar person.

Patty Duke is a celebrity who has been diagnosed as bipolar one. In her book and on her website she does a very good job of explaining the bipolar condition. She tells how she almost lost her family and her career as an actor and actually her life. If you are wondering what level of bipolar is the worst or the best, the answer is there is no better or worse. Every level of bipolar one through eleven has its own unique characteristics and each one is as severe as of all the rest. As an example of bipolar level ten, this person spends most of their time in the depressive side of bipolar. This diagnosis is usually depression. This can be so severe that they will not go outside. They will not answer the phone and will lock themselves in their room and watch TV for days at a time. This would sound like chronic depression, which it is, but it is caused by the bipolar condition. As another example, bipolar one will spend most of their time in the manic state and a very small amount of time in the depressive state. There is no better, best, or worst. They are all part of this hideous mental illness.

The interview that I have to do will be very painful for the victim and me. Adrian has already told me that I am trying to hide all my problems with the bipolar condition. She has said that everyone is crying bipolar. It may seem that way because forty-five percent of the people who are bipolar are not diagnosed. This estimate is based on information from my psychiatrist and the medical community. As stated earlier in this book, only a Psychiatrist can diagnose the bipolar condition. I can say for sure that it runs deep in our family along with other mental conditions.

This may be a good place to explain the need for the human being to alter their brain chemistry and escape by means of alcohol. You might think that alcohol has only been around a short time or maybe since the Roman Empire, not true. The history of alcohol actually dates as far back as 10,000 years BC. This alcohol was discovered from food that had fermented. After eating the food, the Stone Age people got high. They did not know how to explain what happened to them but they did repeat this. India discovered alcohol from wine they made. This dates back to 3000 BC – 2000BC. However this wine was very potent and had very high alcohol content, compare to cheap vodka today. China had discovered alcohol in 7000BC. Persia discovered alcohol in 5400BC – 5000BC. The Roman Empire, along with Egypt, had their own wine from fermenting grapes many thousands of years before current time. This wine had alcohol content higher than our liquor has today. Some of this alcohol had killed people or damaged their brain for the rest of their lives. This, however, did not stop people from drinking the alcohol. Does this sound familiar to you? There have been alcoholics since the discovery of alcohol many thousands of years ago. Why do I bring this up now? Well for many thousands of years we have been trying to alter our brain.

Now do you suppose that our mental illnesses are new to us? No, they are not! I was born with a chemical imbalance in my brain I did not catch it from someone. History shows that mental illness has been around since the beginning of time. In most cases, people were thought to be mad or crazy. Some of these people were killed out of fear, others were cast aside to live their lives alone and to die without help from anyone. I have been told by my doctors that my mental illness has been affecting people forever. Some of our treatments for mental illness over the past fifty years sound like what people did many thousands of years ago. We are now more humane for treating the mentally ill. Shock treatment has long since ended, a very inhumane way of treating the mentally ill. Frontal lobotomy was thought to cure the mentally ill, an extremely cruel treatment practiced in the last 50 years. Today we do not have to worry about being treated like this. We as a society have come a long way in treating and understanding the mentally ill and the bipolar condition.

The Interview

My first wife, Adriane Corday, was the first person whom I interviewed about living with a person who is suffers from bipolar disorder. We were married in 1972 and divorced six years later in1978. At the time we were married, Adriane was seventeen years old and I was twenty-one. Adriane expressed to me that she feels people use the bipolar condition to excuse the terrible things they do. Unfortunately, there are people who use bipolar as an excuse. In my experience, that is not the norm and I have found very few people who do this. I believe it is better to let a hundred criminals go free than to put the wrong person in prison or to death. My goal is that my life story will help people to understand mental illness and bipolar. The following transcript is of the interview I conducted with my first wife. To help in making the dialogue clear, I have transcribed the interview as a third person.

Interviewer: "What was it like to live with someone who is bipolar?"

Adriane: "It was insane; our lifestyle was completely abnormal. I didn't realize how abnormal at first. I was seventeen years old when we married. I trusted Dominick because he was older than I. That was a big mistake. Our marriage was a disaster."

Interviewer: "When did you realize that something was wrong in your marriage?"

Adriane: "I didn't at first. It was exciting for me. It was like a whirlwind that never ended. I was raised to be very responsible and not take chances. Our marriage was never ending parties in bars and at home. I began to believe that this was normal and how young people lived. I watched Dominick destroy things that didn't work right. I saw a lot of rage come out of him and at times, this scared me. He had an incredible temper and sometimes it was directed toward me. Dominick was never physically abusive but he was mentally abusive."

Interviewer: "I know that there was a lot of hurt and pain involved with this. Did you feel that the bipolar person did things to deliberately hurt you? Was this premeditated?"

Adriane: "Yes, I hate him for what he did to me. He used being bipolar as an excuse for his behavior. I believe he did deliberately hurt me. He didn't care how I felt about the wife swapping or anything else we did. We took a lot of acid and partied all the time. He was irresponsible and without feelings for others. I don't believe Dominick knew how to love, doesn't know what love is, or even cares."

Interviewer: "In the time that you were married, was there anything that you could have done differently to stop his behavior?"

Adriane: "No. How could I? I was a young girl. I didn't know what to do. Even when I realized how wrong everything was, there was nothing I could have done. I couldn't control him; no one could. My parents told me to get away from him but I couldn't. I loved him. I could say Dominick ruined my life and at the time, I was helpless to stop him. As I said, I hate him for what he did to me and my family. Dominick never mentioned in the book that I got pregnant with his brother's baby and had to get an abortion. This was the result of the crazy swapping parties we had."

Interviewer: "At any time in this relationship, did you notice mood swings from manic to depressive? If so, what did this look like to you?"

Adriane: "At first, no; I didn't. I began to realize later in our marriage that he was up one minute and down the next. I didn't know at the time he had mental problems. He can hide behind bipolar, but he is insane and should be locked up. Dominick would be depressed and bummed out when things didn't go his way. I think many people hide behind bipolar. Manic was what his life was all the time. He is insane trust me."

Interviewer: "Did your husband go from one thing to another and another without accomplishing anything?"

Adriane: "Yes, It was hard to keep up with him. He would go into many different things at once and most were not completed. He would get bored with one thing and go to another."

Interviewer: "Did your husband do things that were very risky? Did he talk you into doing things that were risky?"

Adriane: "Yes, that was what our lives were based; on being risky .We did things without any planning. He was very spontaneous and that led to an exciting life at first but ended in tragedy."

Interviewer: "Did his risky behavior excite you? If it did, was it a turn on for you?"

Adriane: "At first it was, but then I was only seventeen. The excitement of just picking up and going to New York was something I had never done. The decision to just pick up and go back to California was also. However, this never ended with him."

Interviewer: "I know that drugs and alcohol were a big factor in your husband's life how did this effect you? Since you married at seventeen, did you enjoy the drugs and alcohol for the first time?"

Adriane: "The drinking age was twenty-one in California. When we went to New York, the drinking age was eighteen at that time. That was a whole other thing. I never had the chance to hangout in bars before. Going to the clubs for dancing and drinking was great. The drugs were always around even before we met, but they became a bigger part of our life as time went by. They soon became a problem in our marriage."

Interviewer: "Was there a time in your marriage that you felt threatened, unsafe, or feared your husband? Was there any physical abuse?"

Adriane: "No, I can say that he never hit me or abused me physically. That wasn't what Dominick was all about. His life was always based on fun and enjoyment."

Interviewer: "How do you feel now after many years of divorce?"

Adriane: "My whole life was changed because of Dominick. I feel that my life would have been much different or better without him. That's it that's all I have to say."

Back to September 2010

I was not able to find work in Portland, so I decided to create my own job. I called the True Soda owner in Portland, but he had gone out of business. However, I did find the new person who had bought the franchise in Portland, as well as Seattle. I called him to ask if we could meet. We set a time. Then I went to his warehouse to meet him. His name was Stan. I explained my situation and the business that I had, True Soda in Spokane. I offered to sell soda beverages for him on commission only. That was the only way I would sell anything. I could always make much more money that way. We reached an agreement, and I went to sell the products.

Stan never knew that I was homeless. After we got to know each other and had talked over lunch and beer, both of us opened up. He told me that he would have never known that I was homeless unless I had told him. I found out that he too, had been homeless at one time. After that, we developed a great respect for each other.

This is where some very good things started to happen for me. By this time, I had reached the age of retirement and I retired collecting $1100 a month from Social Security. I remember being homeless and realized that I could retire at the age of sixty-two. I went to the Social Security Office and filed for my retirement. I applied five months before my sixty-second birthday.

I knew that there was a light at the end of this very long tunnel and that is what kept me going. This was when life turned around for me. My goal at this point was to leave the country and live in Mexico, Belize, Costa Rica, or Puerto Rico; anywhere but here. With the money I brought in from retirement I could live very well in any of these places. My lifestyle would consist of a very nice home to live in. I would have a gardener, maid and be able to live the lifestyle that I want by the ocean with the warm sun shining down on me almost every day. Since my passion is motorcycles, I need to live in a climate where I can ride motorcycles most of the year. Portland is not that place.

As God would have it, I found out that I have cysts on my liver and colon and the Hepatitis C has hurt my liver. I know better than anyone that my lifestyle caused a lot of this damage. However, I have also been told that I am a Gnome 2 as far as my DNA goes. What that means is that my liver likely fought off this virus for 26 years. If my life style had been different, I probably would go on for many more years. I have chronic liver disease. If I stop drinking now and take the Interferon treatment, which is 26 weeks of injections, I may live 5 years or more. This is a rough treatment and it's like

Chemo. I have also found out that my autoimmune system is failing. I may not be able to have the Interferon because of my autoimmune system. I could die from the treatment. My autoimmune system failure is not due to AIDS or HIV. In a healthy person the autoimmune system attacks infections and fights off many things that would normally hurt us. Autoimmune System failure simply means that my immune system is attacking my own body trying to hurt me. This could result in Rheumatoid Arthritis or a number of different problems. This disease can attack the liver and further destroy my liver. This disease can also attack the kidneys and cause death.

I have a 60% chance of living five years or more with the Interferon treatment. If I don't I have the treatment I'll have a 10% chance of living anything like five years.

Since I learned that I might not have very long to live I want to enjoy the time I have left. This becomes a very personal choice. Do I want to take the treatments? I now have that choice. The question is what kind of quality of life do I want? For me, that's a no brainer. As you have read in this book, I had lived many lifetimes. I have reinvented myself over and over. At this point, I can't think of anything that I have missed. I have traveled the world and I have taken all the risks that I can think of. I have lived a life that most people only read about.

From Rich to Poor

I have been a millionaire and lost a million dollars. I know what it's like to live in a half a million dollar home and have all the toys that I ever wanted. I know that money does not buy you happiness. What money does buy is freedom of choice. Freedom of choice is very important. It's the difference between living and just getting by. Freedom of choice is waking up one day and deciding that you want to go on a cruise or maybe go to Egypt to see the pyramids. Freedom of choice is what kind of car do I want to drive? That is what I'm talking about. Freedom of choice it is the only thing that money ever did for me. After we lost all that money, it didn't bother me because it was just another adventure; a new chapter in my life.

Losing this money completely devastated Delarosa. The difference between Delarosa and I is that she lived for the money. I lived for what money could buy me; freedom of choice. When our marriage ended, Delarosa threw me out of our home and kept everything. This is how I became homeless. I left with only my clothes. I could have gone after her for half of everything, but I didn't. I suppose one reason was that I knew money meant more to her than anything else in the world. Another reason is I felt incredible guilt over her losing her investment in our business. Most importantly, I have to feel good in my own skin. How would I feel if she were to die tomorrow? I'm sure most everyone who reads this would think I'm insane for not going after half of everything we had.

The truth is that despite everything I have done in my life, I'm a very sensitive person. Maybe I am too sensitive for my own good. The statistics show that a decade ago 95% of all the people in the United States would retire and have only their Social Security to depend on. The statistics also show that only 5% of the population of the United States will ever have over one million dollars. That percentage drops to less than one percent who will have one million dollars at two different times in their lives. Therefore, I Dylan said it best when he said, "If you're not busy living, you're busy dying." Believe me, I was always busy living.

I have great faith in the new generation. I know they will do well; even better than my generation. I believe 95% of all the people in the US are good people do the right thing and follow the law. The other 5% of the population are bad people and don't follow the law. This is expectable in our society. It would be nice to have only 1% of the population who commit crimes but we are not there yet. Some other countries have a much higher crime rate, while some countries have a lower crime rate. Sometimes it seems that what is reported by television, radio and the newspapers is overwhelmingly negative. I attribute this to our instantaneous reporting around the world. The media makes you think that 50% of all the people are bad. When a crime is committed in New York, the west coast knows about it within minutes.

Things may seem worse than they are, but the 95% rule still applies. When I was young, people looked at me and said "These hippies are going ruin the earth, our great country will fall victim to drugs and our system will fail." What did they know? I read some headlines just recently and I will tell you what they said. "There are too many people on the earth; the earth cannot support all of the population.", "Many will starve in the U.S. and many will die.", "The price of everything keeps going up we can't afford much more of this.", "The gas fumes from the autos will kill us all.", "We are in a great inflationary time and if things don't change now we will be in a depression.", "The prisons are filled!" Ominous words in the headlines. I would have feared for my life reading these headlines. However, not to worry these headlines were in the New York Times through the year 1912. This has been going on since the beginning of time. That is why I have faith in the next generation of beautiful people. We will plant trees under which we will never sit and so will they. We will do all the right things and so will they. With a positive attitude and the willingness to change, this generation will overcome. Today there are more doctors graduating from college than ever before. There are more lawyers that will become Judges and take on our legal system. There are more scientists and more trades people in college than ever before.

If you believe like I do, and believe in God; you are half way there. Believe in yourself and our system and you are three quarters there. Believe in the people of the future and you're there. It's going to happen anyway. It always has. Another piece of advice is to remember is there is no one better than anyone else based on what they do. This is hard for people to get their heads around. Certainly, a doctor is a better person than a cook or a waitress. No! Let me say it again, there is no one better than anyone else based on what they do. Think about this for a minute. Have you not heard of some of the things doctors have done? Things that were illegal. We have all heard of corrupt CEO's who embezzled millions from their Corporations. I could go considered myself very lucky to have lived the life that I had. I think Bob Dylan said it best when he said, "If you're not busy living, you're busy dying." Believe me, I was always busy living.

I have great faith in the new generation. I know they will do well; even better than my generation. I believe 95% of all the people in the US are good people do the right thing and follow the law. The other 5% of the population are bad people and don't follow the law. This is expectable in our society. It would be nice to have only 1% of the population who commit crimes but we are not there yet. Some other countries have a much higher crime rate, while some countries have a lower crime rate. Sometimes it seems that what is reported by television, radio and the newspapers is overwhelmingly negative. I attribute this to our instantaneous reporting around the world. The media makes you think that 50% of all the people are bad. When a crime is committed in New York, the west coast knows about it within minutes.

Things may seem worse than they are, but the 95% rule still applies. When I was young, people looked at me and said "These hippies are going ruin the earth, our great country will fall victim to drugs and our system will fail." What did they know? I read some headlines just recently and I will tell you what they said. "There are too many people on the earth; the earth cannot support all of the population.", "Many will starve in the U.S. and many will die.", "The price of everything keeps going up we can't afford much more of this.", "The gas fumes from the autos will kill us all.", "We are in a great inflationary time and if things don't change now we will be in a depression.", "The prisons are filled!" Ominous words in the headlines. I would have feared for my life reading these headlines. However, not to worry these headlines were in the New York Times through the year 1912. This has been going on since the beginning of time. That is why I have faith in the next generation of beautiful people. We will plant trees under which we will never sit and so will they. We will do all the right things and so will they. With a positive attitude and the willingness to change, this generation will overcome. Today there are more doctors graduating from college than ever before. There are more lawyers that will become Judges and take on our legal system. There are more scientists and more trades people in college than ever before.

If you believe like I do, and believe in God; you are half way there. Believe in yourself and our system and you are three quarters there. Believe in the people of the future and you're there. It's going to happen anyway. It always has. Another piece of advice is to remember is there is no one better than anyone else based on what they do. This is hard for people to get their heads around. Certainly, a doctor is a better person than a cook or a waitress. No! Let me say it again, there is no one better than anyone else based on what they do. Think about this for a minute. Have you not heard of some of the things doctors have done? Things that were illegal. We have all heard of corrupt CEO's who embezzled millions from their Corporations. I could go on and on with this, but that is not necessary. What would life be like without cooks and waitresses? Without maids for the hotels or service people who repair our cars. I can tell you now that we need these people in our lives. What about the illegal immigrants who pick our fruit and vegetables in the hot sun all day for minimum wages?

These people do jobs that most of us do not want to do, especially for minimum wages. So the next time you go out for a drink or dinner look at the people who are helping you. Are they worth less than anyone else? Are they worth less than you? Then give them a big smile and compliment them. They deserve it. We get in our own way and forget that we are all equal in God's eyes. The same is true for people who are handicapped or have a mental illness of any kind. Does God punish people for being handicapped? I would hope not. Then we too, should be able to except people who have a handicap. Being bipolar is a very serious handicap.

I never wanted my life to turn out like it did. I didn't try to sabotage myself. I am a very proud man. Does anyone think that I would purposely do this to myself? Most of my life I thought that God hated me and I didn't know why. I always wanted to be like everyone else. Maybe even better, but I didn't know why I couldn't be. I didn't know I had a mental problem. Perhaps if I had, then at least I would have known why I made the choices I did. The times that I was in jail, I had plenty of time to think about myself. I cried for hours and I hated myself. All I wanted was to die. No one but another bipolar or a psychiatrist would understand the pain and loneliness I felt.

That was especially true when I would be in the depressive state. Then that's when I really seen just how screwed up I really was. I was completely hopeless without any way out and I did it to myself. When I wanted to see who did this to me I would look in a mirror. I totally and completely understand why people kill themselves. There have been times when I wanted that more than anything in the world. Just to make the pain go away. Anyone who is bipolar lives in their own private hell. They don't need to be punished. They punish themselves. My psychiatrist has told me that everyone who is bipolar has gone through the same things that I have. That was hard for me to believe. I thought I was the only one in the world who was so screwed up. Maybe the reason why I am still alive is to write this book. There is a bright side to all of this and that is bipolar is the only mental illness that we can treat with medication. We can't cure it at this time, but we can help people live a more normal life. We can help people before they reach the point that I have. That is what this book is all about. If you suspect that you or anyone you know might be bipolar, please take the time to find out.

There are many good websites out there that offer free tests to find out if anyone maybe bipolar. There are many mental health professionals that can and will help. This is a serious matter and it makes the difference between a good happy life and a life which is hell on earth. The younger people are, the harder it may be to admit they have a mental problem. They may never admit it to themselves, you, or anyone else. These young people are the most vulnerable because of the denial associated with Bipolar Disorder or any mental illness.

It is up to us now we are the adults we can make a difference. It takes a lot of love, understanding, and caring. Don't give up on them or yourself. This story of my life is not glamorous. It is sad. My story represents a person losing his whole life for no apparent reason and winding up with nothing. I believe God played a big role in all of this. My strong belief in God can and has pulled me up from the gutters and saved me from a living hell. I have had doctors who told me that the only cure for the personality disorder is God. In addition, they say they have seen God actually cure people from this hideous mental condition.

I have seen young people who have been raised Christian and I see the nice wonderful life they live and will continue to live. When it comes to education and becoming the person that they want to be they have a great head start. Whether they become doctors, surgeons, scientist, or teachers they are miles ahead of the rest. It is the dream of all good parents to believe that their children will grow up and become successful and live the good life. My hope is we will do this for our children's future. Teach them about God and help them when they need it and see that they have a better chance than we did. What do I want now out of life? It's very simple. I want to give back. I want to help people. I want to make people happy and give anything I have to help them. I can't take anything with me when I go, so why not give to others. That is all I want to do now. This thought is what makes me happy!

I also want to bring people to Jesus Christ our Lord and savior. As humans we always want to control everything in our lives. The truth is that we cannot control anything. When we think we are in control, we always lose and never win. I know what you must be thinking. Perhaps you are saying to yourself, "I have controlled my own life and I did very well at it. I have a great family and a great life." Then ask yourself these questions. Am I truly happy with my life? Do I feel that I am satisfied with my life or am I going through life feeling that this is all there is to life? Do I feel truly happy and fulfilled? Is my life filled with joy each day?

Most people I know have simply accepted the life they have. Many of them are very dissatisfied and not really happy at all. Many people live a life of true unhappiness. They do not realize that life could be much better. "Letting go and letting God" is very hard for anyone to do because it means giving up control. Once we turn our lives over to God everything changes for the better. A peace and joy comes over us that many have never experienced. You can see this in the people who have accepted Jesus. They have a glow about them. They are happy. They smile and laugh and enjoy life. You can see it in their eyes. It is said that the eyes are the windows to the soul; then it follows that we can see the soul. When people accept Jesus as their Lord and Savior, it is as if a great weight is lifted from your shoulders.

This is not to say that they do not have all of the same problems as everyone else does. However, all their problems are turned over to Jesus and the burden they carry leaves. In its place is a peace and joy that only God can give. I may not have very long to live, but I am at peace with this. I have not cried over this because I am at peace with God and I know he is there for me. I should be sad, but I am not. One would think that I would live in fear if dyeing, but I do not. Why? That is simple I have turned my life over to God. I am in His hands now, not mine. I may have done many evil things in my life and I have sinned. Jesus died on the cross for my sins and because of that all my sins have been forgiven. This is not to say that I can continue to sin and expect God to forgive me, it doesn't work that way. All God ever wanted from us is to have faith in Jesus and try to live the best life that we can. For God, it's really that simple. The rewards are incredible. I refer to the Bible as the owner's manual for the human being. We did not come with an owner's manual. The Bible teaches us how to live a great and rewarding life. The Bible tells us how to raise our children. The Bible also explains what life will be like when we die. The only requirement for all of this is to except Jesus Christ and try to live the best life that we can. We have to have faith in Jesus and trust that He will take care of us. If you ever wondered what heaven may be like, then I encourage you right now, at this very moment to except Jesus Christ as your Lord and Savior and repent your sins to the Lord. Watch what happens. It is just that simple. Is this too simple to be true? Then give it a try and you see for yourself. What do you have to lose? You have to be very honest when you do this and it has to come from your heart and soul. Once it is done you will see what I am writing about here. This has never failed anyone anywhere in the world and it won't fail you. You will feel a great and wonderful feeling come over you. Faith and trust is all you need. This is the covenant that the Lord has with us. God loves us all and wants us to be with him.

I will supply my email address to you. I want to hear from you and what happens when you turn your life over to Jesus. Please feel free to contact me at daviddominick@yahoo.com and share with me the greatest reward in life; God's love and forgiveness. God bless and have a wonderful life.

My Message to you

As crazy as this may sound, I stopped taking my meds for a couple of months. I guess I missed the high of being manic or maybe I wanted to see if this entire nightmare was really true. Let me tell you that this is the worst thing I've ever done in my life. As a result of not being regulated by my medication, I hurt someone I care about dearly. I hurt them verbally, mentally, and emotionally. I have never experienced the kind of hurt I caused this person and myself. There is no excuse for this. This hurt that I caused haunts me day and night. I can't even imagine anything worse than this.

If any good could come out of that experience, it is that I will never hurt anyone like this again. I pray that this person has a wonderful and happy life for they deserve it. I am sorry more than anyone could ever imagine. The final thing I can share is that over time, my bipolar disorder did get worse. Left untreated, much worse; it's too late for me now. However, it may not be for you. Learn from my mistakes. If you are or know anyone who is diagnosed bipolar and they are prescribed meds, please never stop taking your meds. NEVER. No matter what. This hideous mental illness is the worst thing anyone could ever experience.

"Life is a drawing without an eraser".

God Bless and May you have a wonderful life.

Dominick Delarosso.

About The Author

Dominick Delarosso was born in poverty in Brooklyn, New York. He
lived many lifetimes. Not knowing he was bipolar he lived a very
destructive life. There was no help for him as a child or adult.
Dominick took many people through an exciting life style
And destroyed relationships and people along the way. His
Life is a testament to not only survive but to win in the end.
He was diagnosed bipolar at 58 years old. Dominick
accepted Jesus as his savior and from that moment on he
was changed into a different person. Dominick has said
that the reason he lives today is because of God wanting
him to write this book. He did not live the
life he wanted but he lived the life that God
wanted for him. He has a purpose for everyone
and it might not be what you want
but it will be what God wants.

www.ingramcontent.com/pod-product-compliance
Lightning Source LLC
Chambersburg PA
CBHW060207290526
45789CB00003B/1190